ADVANCED STRATEGY
FOR MEDICAL PRACTICE LEADERS
HUMAN RESOURCES MANAGEMENT EDITION

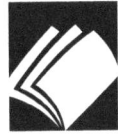

PENNY CROW
MS, RHIA, SHRM-SCP

CHRISTINE KALISH
MBA, CMPE

ANDY SWANSON
MPA, FACMPE

CRISTY GOOD
MPH, MBA, CMPE, CPC

Inspiring
healthcare
excellence.℠

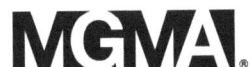

MGMA
104 INVERNESS TERRACE EAST
ENGLEWOOD, CO 80112-5306
877.275.6462
MGMA.COM

MGMA.

Medical Group Management Association® (MGMA®) publications are intended to provide current and accurate information and are designed to assist readers in becoming more familiar with the subject matter covered. Such publications are distributed with the understanding that MGMA does not render any legal, accounting, or other professional advice that may be construed as specifically applicable to individual situations. Neither representations nor warranties are made concerning the application of legal or other principles discussed by the authors to any specific factual situation, nor is any prediction made concerning how any particular judge, government official, or other person will interpret or apply such principles. Specific factual situations should be discussed with professional advisors.

Editors, Bonnie Barnett, Susan Perry, PhD and Andrew Stonehouse, MA

Published by: Medical Group Management Association (MGMA) Library of Congress Control Number: 2022905959

Item: 1047
ISBN: 978-1-56829-026-3

Printed in the United States of America

10 9 8 7 6 5 4 3 2 1

Advanced Strategy for Medical Practice Leaders

Volume 1: Financial Management Edition

Volume 2: Human Resources Management Edition

Volume 3: Operations Management Edition

Contents

Contributors

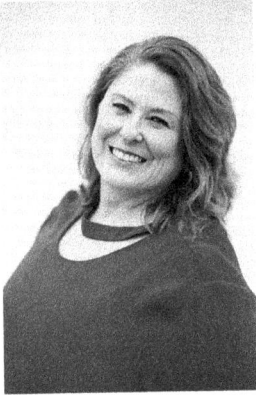

Penny M. Crow, MS, SHRM-SCP, RHIA, is a nationally recognized executive with progressive senior leadership experience in a wide range of healthcare organizations. As an RHIA, she has a successful track record in health information management, revenue cycle, risk management and quality improvement. Her MS in I-O Psychology has fueled her passion about working with leaders to develop strategic thinking skills.

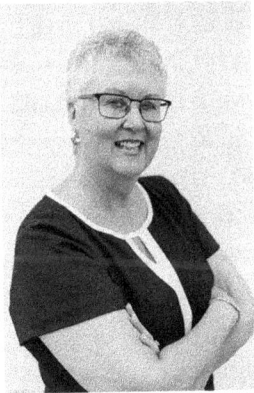

Christine Kalish, MBA, CMPE, is a senior executive and trusted healthcare advisor with deep experience in ambulatory care and academic medicine. She is a thought leader and strategist for emerging and expanding healthcare organizations. For more than thirty years, Kalish has been leading organizations and teams to develop critical infrastructure and growth planning to improve operations, workflow, human resources and revenue cycle. She continually searches for innovative ways to assist her clients so they can deliver quality care for the populations they serve.

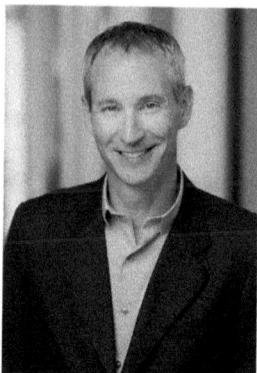

Andy Swanson, MPA, FACMPE, MGMA Senior Vice President of Product Strategy and Sales, has been with MGMA for nine years in a multitude of leadership roles and has spent 18 years inside the human resources function as a daily practitioner, business partner and functional leader. He also brings 13 years of experience in the U.S. healthcare system, both in hospital systems and medical group management. Currently, Swanson deploys products and services for the medical practice industry to improve the people and systems we use to deliver care successfully. Swanson began his career in change management and business consulting, working at Anderson Consulting/Accenture to develop HR solutions around training and development, performance management, compensation, and recruiting and onboarding. Later in the telecommunications and financial services industries, Swanson expanded his expertise by delving into advanced HR strategies, where he led succession planning, leadership development and retention programs for a large regional health system.

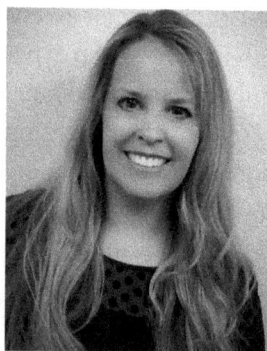

Cristy Good, MPH, MBA, CPC, CMPE, Senior Industry Advisor at MGMA, has expertise in practice management, healthcare operations, revenue cycle management and project management. She has more than 20 years of experience in medical practice administration and financial management. Prior to joining MGMA, Cristy was a credentialed trainer with EPIC and helped prepare providers for one of the largest EHR implementations. For more than five years, she was an administrator with a large health system where she oversaw the strategic and daily operations for multiple outpatient medical practices and also spent six months working for a private home health agency. In addition, she has more than 10 years of clinical laboratory experience.

Special thanks are extended to the following contributors who lent their expertise and insights:

Dawn Plested, JD, MBA, FACHE, Healthcare Management Consultant with MGMA

Marie Eslick, Human Resources Director at Apex Dermatology and Skin Center in Concord, Ohio

Tony Schirer, MBA, FACMPE, Executive Director of Cheyenne OBGYN

Introduction

This is the second book in MGMA's *Advanced Strategy for Medical Practice Leaders* series. *Volume 1: Financial Management Edition*, covered best financial practices that can help optimize revenue cycle integrity and minimize costs for healthcare organizations. *Volume 3: Operations Management Edition* will conclude this series as it explores the many aspects of overall administrative operations and structures for medical practices. This book, the *Human Resources Management Edition*, looks at how modern medical group practices can integrate human resource strategies to improve the employment lifecycle and organizational culture. It endeavors to explore the many facets of HR management strategies within the context of the healthcare industry while allowing that these strategies can vary from one practice to another. Wherever applicable, it is incumbent upon the reader to use this guide as a template and place it within the context of their organization.

This book will first cover how strategic planning can align HR's goals with the organization's overall business needs while fostering effective communication and promoting a positive organizational culture. Next, it explores all aspects of the employment lifecycle from pre-employment to separation. It will also go in depth about job analysis, compensation benefits design, the strategic use of key performance indicators (KPIs) to measure and optimize HR processes, as well as the importance of complying with federal labor laws. We will also hear directly from healthcare experts as they give insights into applying these strategies with examples from their experiences.

Forward-thinking groups are working from the perspective of what means the most to their staff while enabling them to best serve patients. To accomplish this, medical practices are thinking about each stage of the employee lifecycle within their group and how they can best meet employee needs while meeting the needs of both the practice and patients. We will examine human resources management processes (tools, procedures and best practices) while providing examples of applying these concepts within a healthcare setting. While offering a model of effectively deploying these strategies, each chapter emphasizes overarching themes of improving leadership, better managing staff and creating a safe and diverse workplace culture.

This book assumes a dedicated HR role or function within a medical practice. For those medical groups, it is intended to dive into great depth to ensure that their HR practices emulate or exceed the best practices for employees. For those groups without a dedicated HR function and for lead administrators reading this book seeking guidance about employing strategic HR, fear not. It is possible to commit to strategic people leadership, align with the organization's physicians and stakeholders, and deploy many of the core concepts presented even without a dedicated HR leader. It is possible to set a practice apart by using this book as a guideline to deploy exemplary aspects of HR leadership without making HR a full-time job and while still wearing the many hats of small-practice administration.

By applying the strategies and concepts outlined in this book, HR professionals and healthcare leaders will be better equipped to navigate the complexities of their roles, drive organizational growth and create a positive and engaging work environment.

Chapter 1

Strategic Planning for HR Professionals

1.1 Strategic Planning

In today's changing healthcare landscape, strategic human resources planning is important for ensuring organizational success and sustainability. This chapter explores the importance of strategic planning in healthcare HR, various strategic planning models, aligning strategic planning with business needs, the transition from business intelligence to business analytics and the major challenges facing the healthcare industry.

Why a Strategic Plan?

Strategic planning involves a systematic process of setting goals, objectives, and action plans to meet the organization's workforce needs and support its mission and vision. It encompasses forecasting future workforce requirements through the use of data analytics, identifying talent gaps, and developing strategies to recruit, retain and develop a skilled workforce. Medical Group Management Association (MGMA) encourages its leaders to make this plan a useful living document. As healthcare consultant Owen Dahl, MBA, LFACHE, CHBC, LSSMBB, says, a strategic business plan "will always help you keep a focus on your priorities and clarify your direction as you move forward ... The more you commit to the planning process, the more you will also be committed to your goals."[1] Strategic planning can offer a roadmap to key decisions made within the organization.

HR's Role in Strategic Planning

HR plays a crucial role in strategic planning in a healthcare organization. They contribute their expertise in human resources management to align the organization's workforce with its strategic goals and objectives. Some key areas where HR's involvement is essential include workforce planning and talent management, organizational development and change management, performance management and metrics, leadership development and succession planning, and employment engagement and communication.

From 2021-2022, tens of millions of American workers left their jobs in what is dubbed The Great Resignation. *Newsweek* reported on U.S. Bureau of Labor statistics that ranked healthcare among the industries hit hardest, losing more than 500,000 employees per month in 2022 alone.[2] Although staffing has historically been an ongoing issue in healthcare, The Great Resignation further added the need for HR professionals and healthcare leaders to find strategic solutions to hiring and retaining a talented workforce. Although this book will discuss staffing, strategic staffing and various staffing models will be further explored in *Operations Management*, the next edition of the *Advanced Strategy for Medical Practice Leaders* series.

Strategic planning is a collaborative process. It is during this process when multiple perspectives can be considered.

- How does the practice appear to those from outside?
- What does a patient see?
- What do employees see?
- What do applicants see?
- What does the community see?

How the strategic plan is communicated helps with buy-in from the providers and staff. Effective communication requires good listening skills. It is critical to listen to the objections of the providers and staff to allow mitigation before formally announcing the new direction. It is essential that each team member knows and understands the "why" of a strategy. It may only sometimes persuade naysayers to change positions, but understanding the "why" gains support. Sometimes the support is more important than the consensus for an idea.

The strategic plan is only as valuable as the strategic thinking used to develop it. The strategy must be flexible and directional all at the same time. Finally, the strategy will provide clear guidance on allocating time and resources for HR and the staff.

1.2 Strategic Planning Aligns with Business Needs

Once the organization has provided the direction, the strategic human resource leader can identify the skills that will be needed by asking:

- Who among the current staff has the required skills?
- Is a focused recruitment strategy needed?
- What training needs to happen to bridge the gap from the current experience level to upskilling for the future direction?

Strategy is the decision-making tool that will help determine the path taken. It is a roadmap that will help assess focus, goals and direction. Strategic HR is the way to demonstrate that HR is a trusted resource in the practice and understands where the organization is going. Most large organizations have already identified the need and value of a strategic HR leader, but unfortunately, small and medium-sized businesses have room to work toward this goal. HR leaders can not only influence employees with direction and a roadmap, but they can also help prepare the staff for executive leadership's strategies.

When the HR director is included as a strategic partner, benefits realized by an organization can include:

- Avoiding costly surprises
- Being proactive to avoid crises
- Increasing staff productivity
- Keeping employees focused on organizational goals and providing strategic training and development of upskilling current clinical and administrative staff

Strategic alignment focuses on results-oriented goals. Examples include:

- Correctly assessing staff and skills
- Developing and maintaining competitive pay and benefits
- Managing performance
- Knowing what the competitors are doing to recruit and retain talent
- Identifying a meaningful reward program

When an organization is considering a new strategy, HR must be able to understand and determine the probable long-term ramifications. Determining the effect of HR decisions before implementing the strategy allows for proactive rather than reactive leadership.

Strategic Planning Models

Several strategic planning models can guide HR professionals in healthcare organizations:

- **SWOT analysis:** Assessing strengths, weaknesses, opportunities, and threats helps identify internal capabilities and external factors influencing HR strategy.
- **PESTLE analysis:** Analyzing political, economic, social, technological, legal, and environmental factors enables HR to anticipate changes and adapt strategies as needed.
- **Balanced Scorecard:** Aligning HR objectives with organizational goals and measuring performance across financial, customer, internal processes, learning and growth perspectives.
- **Scenario Planning:** Creating alternative future scenarios helps HR anticipate potential workforce challenges and develop contingency plans.

In today's healthcare space, it can be helpful for HR professionals to know business basics like finance, marketing, operations and technology. An HR professional must understand budgets, spreadsheets and forecasting. This business understanding will lead to more leadership development and support as an internal coach to help teams manage change.

One way to support the strategic HR process is a "SWOT" analysis. The SWOT analysis should be completed through an objective view or balcony perspective, including a diverse group of staff, not just the usual decision-makers. It's also important to determine what sets your practice apart, and if that brings you strength or may be a threat because others are doing it in your marketplace.[3]

Exhibit 1.1 SWOT Analysis

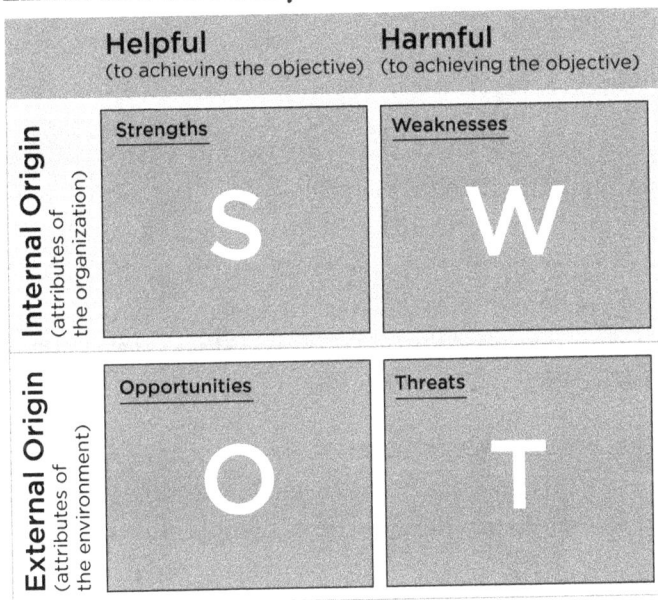

At a minimum, strategic HR should align with the organization's goals for workforce planning, talent development, change management as well as the more contemporary focus on issues of diversity, equity and inclusion (DEI). The Great Resignation forced organizations to analyze goals with available talent, attract new talent or determine if workflow could be restructured to eliminate the need for a job rather than filling a vacancy. According to the Journal of General Internal Medicine, it also suggested it was time to rebuild healthcare business culture to better support the needs of employees, from providers to front-line staff.[4] The use of technology has created a new skill set for employees requiring upskilling resulting in talent development programs.

As well, the high percentage of staff diagnosed with burnout in healthcare has required a different approach to productivity. According to the HHS, excessive workloads, administrative burdens, limited say in scheduling and a lack of organizational support are the biggest factors in burnout; systemic workforce shortages also continue, with an anticipated shortfall of roughly 100,000 physicians by 2033.[5] With five generations in the workplace, numerous ways are necessary to communicate, work and balance life. In many ways, the only thing that provides a competitive advantage is the people.

Transactional HR vs. Strategic HR

In today's marketplace, HR serves as more than merely a transactional function. Transactional HR refers to the operational and administrative activities that are essential for maintaining HR processes within an organization. Encompassing a range of essential tasks that keep HR operations running smoothly, transactional HR includes payroll administration, benefits management, recruitment and onboarding, compliance with labor laws, record-keeping and employee data management.

Strategic HR involves anticipating and supporting the strategic needs of the business. This involves more intangible tasks like proactively identifying workplace development needs, developing performance management processes and implementing effective recruitment and retention strategies.[6]

Regardless of if an organization has a dedicated HR professional, it is necessary to have someone who demonstrates competency when staffing the HR function. The Society for Human Resource Management (SHRM) has identified nine competencies to succeed in strategic HR.[7]

They include:

1. Human resource expertise
2. Relationship management
3. Consultation
4. Leadership and navigation
5. Communication

6. Global and cultural effectiveness

7. Ethical practice

8. Critical evaluation

9. Business acumen

When an organization outsources the daily operations of HR, there should still be an overall HR service delivery plan that integrates the outsourced functions and the internal responsibilities.

Strategic HR professionals will use data analytics to make decisions and recommend specific strategies to support the organization's plan for a successful future.

1.3 Moving from Business Intelligence to Business Analytics

According to a report by Arcadia, a leading data analytics platform for healthcare, only 57% of healthcare organizations use data to make decisions.[8] This could be because, as the *HBR* explains, the size and scale of most healthcare businesses means "there is almost no reason for HR to use the special software and tools associated with big data."[9] However, most organizations do use HR technology to report talent-related data to describe what has happened in the past, a process known as descriptive analytics. In contrast, high-performing HR professionals use statistical models to make predictions for the future and prescriptive analytics for decision-making. Why does this matter? Many HR professionals report that getting to "the table" for critical discussions and strategic decisions is difficult. Those who get a seat at the table have demonstrated that they understand how to measure and report decisions made for the organization's people management and overall business initiatives.

HR's Role with Data

SHRM statistics suggest it takes an average of 42 days to fill an open position, and considerably more if trying to hire healthcare providers and specialists.[10] The Association for Advancing Physician and Provider

Recruitment (AAPPR) performed an *In-House Physician and Provider Recruitment Benchmarking Report* in 2020.[11] The report found that in 2019, recruiters reported it took an average of 123 days to fill a physician search and 63 days for advanced practice providers. In addition, credentialing adds at least another 120 days from hire. With these pre-pandemic figures in mind, organizations today should implement plans on what providers can do during this transition period—otherwise the provider's start date can be postponed until they can see patients.

Metrics such as "time to hire"—the time between the moment your eventual hire entered your pipeline through sourcing and an application, and the moment they accepted your job offer—are important. Monitoring and evaluating this type of data will result in finding roadblocks in processes that may prevent getting the best hires.

As professor and author Peter Cappelli notes in *HBR*, "One of the reasons for the special attention being given to big data in HR is that the department is always under pressure to be more analytic—which is justified to some extent. Some wishful thinkers believe that the application of big data techniques will somehow rid HR of some of the attributes they don't like about it, such as the perception that they're focusing on "soft" issues and not detailing the return on HR-related investments."

Several key performance indicators (KPIs) are commonly used in HR strategy to measure the effectiveness of HR initiatives and their effect on organizational goals. Some of the most common KPIs in HR strategy include:

- Employee Turnover Rate
- Time-to-Fill
- Cost-per-Hire
- Employee Engagement Score
- Training and Development ROI
- Absenteeism Rate
- Performance Appraisal Completion Rate
- Employee Satisfaction
- Revenue per Employee

With all the recent research in healthcare regarding diversity, equality and inclusion, consider measuring its effect on a competitive advantage. How does it affect patient care and outcomes? Are decisions made in a vacuum because differences are not considered? How well is diversity measured in the organization? See Chapter 8 to better understand how metrics can be incorporated into HR strategy.

Data is an essential component of strategic HR decisions. By asking the right questions and focusing on the best ways to collect and present the data, strategic HR professionals can collaborate with leadership in critical decision-making discussions.

Strategic Goals

Utilizing data is crucial for determining an organization's strategic goals, regardless of its size. Taking the initiative to discuss them with executive leadership can help determine direction for growth and competitive advantage. Choose three things the medical practice wants to focus on regarding the competitive advantage. How will the practice differentiate itself from other practices in the market? The reality is that today, practices are competing for patients, providers and staff. Once the organizational strategic goals are determined, it is time to put strategic HR into practice starting with business intelligence. Business intelligence is looking at past and present data to identify trends and explain what has happened with talent management historically to make decisions in the present for day-to-day operations.

Asking questions is vital to data analysis. Once a strategic goal is identified, the first natural questions are:

- How can HR help achieve this goal?
- Which initiatives identified by executive leadership can HR implement?
- What information would be useful to measure the success of these initiatives?

Moving from transactional HR to more strategic HR means using data to predict and forecast future needs based on statistical models. It uses the data to correlate business and people data to improve an organization's performance. As an organization grows, investments in technology and state-of-the-art metrics can allow for more sophisticated strategies.

1.4 Major Challenges Facing the Healthcare Industry

Strategic HR can help healthcare organizations find innovative solutions to the many challenges that affect staffing, culture and quality of care. These solutions not only address the challenges that have surfaced in recent years, but also the challenges that healthcare has always encountered.

The healthcare industry faces numerous challenges that affect HR strategy:

- **Workforce Shortages and Retention:** Addressing shortages of healthcare professionals, including physicians, nurses and allied health workers, requires innovative recruitment and retention strategies.
- **Healthcare Reform:** Adapting to regulatory changes, healthcare reform initiatives, and value-based care models necessitates workforce agility and flexibility.
- **Technological Advancements:** Embracing digital health technologies, telemedicine, and artificial intelligence requires upskilling and reskilling the healthcare workforce.
- **Workforce Well-being:** Supporting employee health and well-being, particularly in high-stress healthcare environments, is essential for workforce morale, engagement and retention.

The ability to find staff will be the greatest struggle for HR professionals in the coming decade, with projections from the U.S. Bureau of Labor Statistics suggesting that more than 200,000 additional nurses will be needed each year to help offset retirement and address demand.[12]

To help address those recruiting issues, healthcare employers can follow the lead of other industries and consider a range of benefits to attract top talent, including:

- Training and advancement opportunities
- Signing bonuses
- Flexible working conditions
- Competitive compensation and benefits packages

Paying attention to wages is also critical, as even service and hospitality employers have raised their rates to attract talent.

For staff who weathered the extended hours and difficult working conditions in clinics and hospitals during the pandemic, burnout came into focus as another key HR issue. "When you're short-staffed in healthcare, the rest of the team takes it on and gets burned out," says Carrie O'Dell, with Group Health Cooperative of South Central Wisconsin. What's more, the nature of healthcare work seems to create a never-ending cycle of fatigue, she adds. "The emotional burnout of taking on everyone else's sicknesses, depersonalizing it, doing it all day, adds up to a different type of burnout than having a lot of work to do."[13]

Being cognizant of that stress—from providers all the way to frontline office staff—can also help shift HR focus to flexibility and benefits that range from more robust paid time off to employee recognition. Improved training, especially in emerging digital technologies, can also reduce the time spent on paperwork and provide more time for patient care for all members of the team.

HR professionals must also cope with the complexities of licensing and compliance to cope with requirements that vary from state to state, which is especially important in multistate healthcare organizations. The emergence of remote work and telehealth flexibility during COVID-19 led to a relaxation of rules regarding residency and licensing, and those changes will continue to impact the way that healthcare is delivered—and the expectations of healthcare employees.[14]

Combined together, the litany of modern challenges require HR professionals to be adept, interactive and inventive in their strategies to help attract, retain and enhance the lives of their employees. They are all issues to be considered as HR works with senior managers to help plan for success.

1.5 Practice in Action

Dayton Children's, a pediatric subspecialist, sought to fulfill their mission that focuses on being the healthcare resource to all children of the Miami Valley regardless of their socioeconomic status. Once physicians are recruited, there is a strong sense of urgency on their part, and the hospital's, to ramp up into a productive and satisfying practice and to begin treating the 290,000 babies, children and adolescents seeking their care through outpatient and inpatient services every year.

Yet, process, policy and communication barriers often delayed the full integration of physicians into their practice. The leadership of Dayton Children's physician services determined that—in addition to the negative effect on access to care—the broken onboarding process was measurably influencing physician engagement, satisfaction and revenue production. There were also unacceptable collateral costs in terms of high turnover and inefficient recruitment, which compounded the lack of access and revenue impact.

With at least 10 different hospital and group practice departments who touch onboarding, Dayton Children's convened an integrated task force to deconstruct the complex process of onboarding new physicians. Through the use of Lean techniques, they rebuilt it to be simpler, more efficient and faster. The framework and consultation established an integrated and rigorous approach to physician onboarding and navigation. Through a rapid improvement event, Dayton completed the identification and removal of barriers and redundancies.

The year-long physician mentorship program, critical to retention, was structured under the direction of their Onboarding Coach and Mentor. Dayton provided physician leadership and representation of the medical staff on the onboarding task force. New physicians and their mentors were matched for compatibility and shared commitment to program goals.

Dayton Children's then implemented a Board Management Software and achieved measurable improvements within the first two years. Their results included a reduction in credentialing time from 322 to 84 days, acceleration in getting physicians working at full productivity from 14 months to 5 months and reduction in turnover from 11.6% to 2.7%.[15]

1.6 Summary

Strategic planning can be a crucial element for any healthcare organization to realize their strategic goals. But the payoff can be a broader and more comprehensive understanding of the issues and challenges facing all levels of staff. By incorporating data analysis into those decisions, HR leaders can make better decisions regarding trends and changes, such as the recent labor market issues in the post-pandemic world.

To summarize, here are some of the key points discussed in this chapter:

- Strategic planning examines the organization's competitive advantage, strengths and areas for improvement. It involves thinking about the organization's path from the short-term to the long-term, being proactive in determining what direction an organization will take. Ultimately, strategic planning defines how to navigate the roadmap to manifest an organization's vision.
- Strategic HR involves more than the standard transactional HR function. It's anticipating and supporting the strategic needs of the business by proactively identifying workplace development needs, developing performance management processes and implementing effective recruitment and retention strategies.
- Moving from transactional HR to more strategic HR means using data to predict and forecast future needs based on statistical models. Utilizing data can be crucial for determining an organization's strategic goals.
- Modern challenges to medical staffing require HR professionals to be adept, interactive and inventive in their strategies to help attract, retain and enhance the lives of their employees. Healthcare employers can follow the lead of

other industries and consider offering a range of benefits from competitive compensation and benefits to advancement opportunities.

- Significant challenges facing healthcare HR include talent acquisition, employee burnout, constant need for retraining and significant changes to laws and licensing requirements. By collaborating with senior managers and practice owners, healthcare HR professionals can address these challenges through improved short-term and long-term planning.

The next chapter will examine how organizational culture and communication can better allow for strategic thinking to come into play for all employees of a modern healthcare practice.

Notes

1. MGMA. https://www.mgma.com/articles/creating-an-optimal-strategic-business-plan
2. Newsweek. https://www.newsweek.com/great-resignation-hits-healthcare-actions-take-1761064
3. MGMA. https://www.mgma.com/articles/creating-an-optimal-strategic-business-plan
4. https://www.ncbi.nlm.nih.gov/pmc/articles/PMC9243774/
5. HHS. https://www.hhs.gov/surgeongeneral/priorities/health-worker-burnout/index.html
6. LinkedIn. https://www.linkedin.com/pulse/evolving-from-transactional-strategic-hr-roadmap-srivastava
7. Steven Darien. https://medium.com/@StevenDarien/the-nine-competencies-of-the-shrm-competency-model-786 22a70def6
8. PR Newswire. https://www.prnewswire.com/news-releases/report-only-57-of-healthcare-organizations-data-is-us ed-to-make-decisions-301886374.html
9. *HBR*. https://hbr.org/2017/06/theres-no-such-thing-as-big-data-in-hr
10. SHRM. https://www.shrm.org/hr-today/news/hr-magazine/spring2020/pages/health-care-industry-top-hr-challenges.aspx
11. AAPPR. https://chghealthcare.com/blog/healthcare-recruiting-trends
12. American Association of Colleges of Nursing. https://www.aacnnursing.org/news-data/fact-sheets/nursing-shortage

13. SHRM. https://www.shrm.org/hr-today/news/hr-magazine/spring2020/pages /health-care-industry-top-hr-challenges.aspx

14. Obsidian HR. https://www.obsidianhr.com/what-you-need-to-know-multi-state -compliance/

15. Tiller-Hewitt. https://www.tillerhewitt.com/case-studies/onboardplus-improves -engagement-productivity-and/

Chapter 2

Organizational Culture and Communication

2.1 Importance of Culture

This chapter will examine how a positive work culture can allow employees to feel valued for their contributions and better connected to their jobs over the long term. We will define culture as well as HR's involvement in strategies to help improve workplace culture through more effective communication and direct interaction with employees. Finally, readers will learn about the increasing focus on diversity, equity and inclusion, and how to better integrate that into a medical organization's daily operations and recruiting efforts.

Creating an influential organizational culture will maximize the success of a medical practice. The American Medical Association (AMA) describes organizational culture as "a set of underlying rules and beliefs that determine how your team interacts with patients and each other."[1] An essential component of this process is a good employee engagement strategy. The more invested employees are, the more productive they will be.

What Defines an Organization's Culture

Regardless of size, a healthcare organization's culture is defined by the expectations, values and practices it instills into all employees. There is no separation between management and staff in organizational culture.

Organizational culture develops best when everyone—from leadership to staff shares similar expectations to promote a positive culture.

An effective, strategic organizational culture is rarely achieved with the "do as I say but not as I do" mindset. A winning, sustainable culture is achieved when employees see that management and employees actively participate in the same manner. As healthcare consultant group Press Ganey says, employee engagement in healthcare begins with a paradigm shift: "Organizations must make strategic decisions in how they think about employee engagement and experience, taking an approach that's inherently more connected and human-centric."[2]

To that end, here are some vital strategic benefits realized from organizational culture improvement:

- Increased employee engagement
- Increased employee satisfaction and productivity
- Core values of the practice are evident in daily operations
- Enhanced teamwork and collaboration
- Improved quality of care and patient satisfaction
- Innovation and continuous improvement
- Stronger organizational reputation

According to a 2023 Gallup survey: company culture and employee engagement work in partnership to ensure the success of any business.[3] A successful workplace culture engages staff, inspires them to do their best and provides comfort to team members. When someone feels valued and part of the team, they are more likely to work harder towards the shared vision and goals. Employees who enjoy their work environment are more likely to stay regardless of salary issues. Engaged employees boost the overall work environment and spread positivity around their coworkers. Also, engaged employees are committed to their jobs and strive to perform their best, resulting in decreased absenteeism and turnover.

Gallup also reports that companies with a high level of employee engagement are also more profitable by an estimated 21%.[4] In contrast, disengaged employees contribute less, lack motivation and decrease overall productivity, costing employers an estimated $450 billion yearly. In an

11-year study for their book, *Corporate Culture and Performance*, John P. Kotter and James Heskett report that companies with positive, influential corporate cultures experienced a 682% growth in revenue.[5] Creating a consistent, positive organizational culture is paramount to building a lasting, prosperous business or medical practice.

Sustaining High-Performance Culture

There are many elements to developing and sustaining a high-performance organizational culture. These include hiring practices, onboarding efforts, recognition programs and performance management programs. Some of the most well-known companies revered for their organizational cultures emphasize employee satisfaction at the root. Some of these organizations offer examples of employee empowerment that can significantly transform the patient experience while enriching the lives of workers.

Ranked number one on Fortune's Best Workplaces in Healthcare, Elevance Health (formerly Anthem, Inc.) serves more than 118 million people through a diverse portfolio of medical, digital, pharmacy, behavioral, clinical and complex care solutions. Roughly 86% of their employees say Elevance Health is a great place to work, compared to 57% of employees at a typical American-based company.[6] Contributing to that employee satisfaction comes from Elevance's partnership with ianacare, an app that combines technology and human-led support for caregivers. After discovering that a large portion of their workforce were caregivers, Elevance Health integrated its already existing benefits and EAP services into ianacare's platform with a goal of bolstering talent retention and advancement while addressing the new ways their associates were integrating their personal life into hybrid work.[7]

Even simple ideas can have a significant boost on employee morale. Benefits like free teeth cleaning for all staff at dental practices can be low-cost employee retention benefits. There is tremendous value in leveraging what is cost-effective with the wants and needs of the team to achieve improved satisfaction rates and longevity. In an MGMA report, strategies such as behavior modeling, better communication, engagement and empowerment for employees were also demonstrated to provide cost-effective ways of shoring up overall organizational culture. "At the end of the day, staff engagement is a willingness to, in every experience, cause a moment of delight," says Debra Wiggs, Founder of V2V Management Solutions. "It's a staff member who walks into their role and responsibility, who identifies whoever their [client] is, with an intention to delight."[8]

EMPLOYEE SATISFACTION SURVEY

[Healthcare Organization Name]

Introduction: Thank you for taking the time to participate in our Employee Satisfaction Survey. Your feedback is essential in helping the HR department understand the needs and concerns of our employees. Your responses are anonymous and confidential.

Section 1: Demographics

Please answer the following questions to help us better understand the composition of our workforce:

* Department/Unit:
  - ☐ Clinical (e.g., nursing, physician)
  - ☐ Non-Clinical (e.g., administration, HR)
  - ☐ Support Services (e.g., maintenance, housekeeping)
* Job Title:
* Years of Service at [Healthcare Organization Name]:

Section 2: Job Satisfaction

Please rate your level of satisfaction with the following aspects of your job on a scale of 1 (very dissatisfied) to 5 very satisfied):

- _____ Workload and Work-Life Balance
- _____ Compensation and Benefits
- _____ Professional Growth and Development Opportunities
- _____ Communication within the Organization
- _____ Supervisor/Manager Support
- _____ Teamwork and Collaboration
- _____ Recognition and Appreciation for Your Work

Section 3: Work Environment

Please indicate your level of agreement with the following statements:

The workplace is safe and conducive to providing quality patient care.

- _____ Strongly Agree
- _____ Agree
- _____ Neutral
- _____ Disagree
- _____ Strongly Disagree

I have the necessary resources and equipment to perform my job effectively.

- _____ Strongly Agree
- _____ Agree
- _____ Neutral
- _____ Disagree
- _____ Strongly Disagree

The organization fosters a culture of respect and diversity.

- _____ Strongly Agree
- _____ Agree
- _____ Neutral
- _____ Disagree
- _____ Strongly Disagree

Section 4: Healthcare Quality and Patient Care

Please rate your level of agreement with the following statements related to healthcare quality:

The care provided to patients at [Healthcare Organization Name] is of high quality.

- _____ Strongly Agree
- _____ Agree
- _____ Neutral
- _____ Disagree
- _____ Strongly Disagree

I have the necessary resources and support to provide excellent patient care.

- _____ Strongly Agree
- _____ Agree
- _____ Neutral
- _____ Disagree
- _____ Strongly Disagree

Inspiring
healthcare
excellence.™

MGMA.

EMPLOYEE SATISFACTION SURVEY (CONTINUED)

Section 5: HR Department and Support

Please share your thoughts on the HR department and its services:

How would you rate your interactions with the HR department in terms of responsiveness and helpfulness?

_____ Excellent

_____ Good

_____ Fair

_____ Poor

Are there any HR-related services or programs you believe could be improved or expanded?

Section 6: Suggestions and Comments

Please provide any additional comments, suggestions, or concerns related to your employment experience or the healthcare organization as a whole.

Remember to analyze the survey results carefully and use the feedback to inform HR initiatives, address concerns, and enhance the overall employee experience in your healthcare organization.

Inspiring
healthcare
excellence.

MGMA.

When dealing with healthcare, it is not always possible to relax the work environment as in other workplace settings. There are safety procedures in place for good reason, but even a small token of appreciation, such as a work-sponsored meal for the staff, goes a long way. During the pandemic, clinics were trying to improve employee morale with weekly office lunches. But over time, the repeated lunches became monotonous and no longer came off as an expression of appreciation. The timing and type of employer-sponsored meals, parties and such need to be varied so that they seem special and help make employees feel appreciated. The unexpectedness of a gesture shows appreciation and promotes positive employee morale. When sharing an employer-sponsored meal is restricted to only holidays, it can often be interpreted as an obligation rather than an actual sign of thanks. Celebrating the staff on anniversaries and birthdays is another small way to appreciate each employee publicly.

Before developing strategies for culture improvement in the practice, keep a few things in mind.

- **The culture should make employees feel valued and comfortable:** No one wants to work in a hostile environment, nor do they want to feel uncomfortable while at work. The workplace needs to be welcoming and structured with clear expectations yet flexible to the growing and changing needs of the staff. Adaptability strategies in culture development will improve success rates.

- **Work with the team to develop consensus:** Define acceptable behavior, standards for employee interaction and core values that promote the best possible work environment while promoting the business. It is recommended to stay within <u>five core values</u>.

- **Communicate, educate and involve employees:** Once the core values are determined, they must be communicated to the entire organization and reinforced by practice leaders through leading by example.

- **Get together often:** Interoffice relationships at every level affect productivity. Leadership needs to be available to the staff for collaborative meetings. These meetings can be informal (town hall style) or more personal (one-on-one).

The goal is to open the door for information to flow both ways. Leaders are responsible for motivating and guiding employees. For an organization to be truly successful, all teams must communicate and collaborate effectively, and it is essential to establish open communication across all departments. Strongly encourage the providers to participate in these gatherings. It takes a village to keep the clinic running smoothly.

When leadership engages with employees or operates with consideration of employees' known wants and desires, the success rate increases. It is essential to be open-minded and adaptable to modifications as the process is implemented and developed over time, and this dedication to the process will ensure success.

Mayo Clinic utilizes a values review process to support and maintain its values.[9] Top leadership at Mayo Clinic supports and encourages time for teams to have values-focused discussions and reflect on how the values are expressed in their work. Reviewers highlight the effect the values have on the entire organization while the institution supports the values-review process by paying for staff time to participate. A values review is a discussion-based virtual or in-person activity that includes the following steps:

Exhibit 2.1 Value Review Process

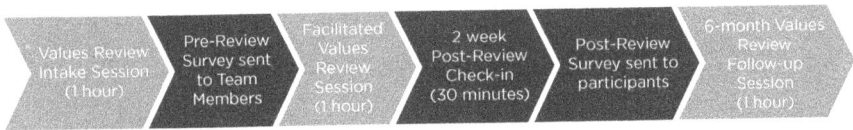

| Values Review Intake Session (1 hour) | Pre-Review Survey sent to Team Members | Facilitated Values Review Session (1 hour) | 2 week Post-Review Check-in (30 minutes) | Post-Review Survey sent to participants | 6-month Values Review Follow-up Session (1 hour) |

A defined organizational culture—in a workplace led by a medical practice administration that can effectively develop its staff through good communication and appropriately aligned incentives—can keep the culture improving over time, benefitting the practice, its employees and its patients. Creating and maintaining exceptional organizational culture is especially important in a healthcare setting, according to MGMA contributor Rosalba Miranda Lozano, BBA, MBA, LLSGB, FACMPE.[10]

"Having the privilege to take care of patients every day is one of the most vital and pivotal lessons learned through working healthcare," she says. "Healthcare organizations must have the right internal culture that keeps providers and staff motivated to perform their best every day; patients deserve world-class care when they trust a particular institution for their well-being."

2.2 Defining Culture

A well-defined organizational culture in the workplace is crucial to motivating staff and promoting the organization's growth. According to Achievers, an employee survey analyst, 77% of employees consider a company's culture before applying, and culture is one of the main reasons 65% of employees stay in their job—almost half of employees would leave their current position for a lower-paying job at a company with better culture.[11]

According to Gallup research:

- Employees with a strong connection to their organization's culture show higher levels of engagement.
- Engaged employees are more likely to refer friends to their organization.
- 71% of workers say that they use referrals from current employees of an organization to learn about job opportunities.

Employee retention strategies to attract and retain highly qualified employees are discussed further in Chapter 6.

Recognition and Reward

According to a 2023 study by Great Place to Work, when employees are given on-the-job recognition, they are 2.2 times more likely to go above and beyond their regular duties. They are also 2.6 times more likely to think that promotions are fair, and 2.2 times more likely to drive innovation and bring new ideas forward.[12] A practice could consider giving various incentives for employees to stay with the company for an extended amount of time.

Here are some examples of incentive programs typically offered:

Tuition reimbursement: Tuition reimbursement for certification and other programs for career development is a mutually beneficial incentive program. Tuition reimbursement is significantly meaningful to those employees that want to advance in the medical field but have minimal or no means to pay for their education. The amount for tuition reimbursement varies from $1,000 to $5,000 and is traditionally only available to employees who have proven loyalty with consistent employment for at least two years.

FSA (Flexible Spending Account): An incentive program especially valued by employees with families is a medical spending account. It acts like a self-funded loan that allows the employee to set aside pre-tax dollars via payroll deductions to an account set up to make medical payments toward copays or any other medical, dental, or vision costs.

Paid time-off: Another incentive option could be as small as offering an additional paid day off on the employee's company service anniversary or birthday every year, as part of a robust overall PTO package. According to SHRM, organizations that also implemented a combined PTO program—banking sick time and vacation time together—found that unscheduled absences dropped by up to 10%. "We made the switch because our people were not using their sick time and were complaining about not having enough time off," says Kerry Wekeolo, of Actualize Consulting. "So we combined it to a total of four weeks' paid time off. Our people love this, and even as we hire new recruits, they rave about starting at a firm with four weeks' vacation."[13]

Onsite gym or low-cost gym membership as a group benefit: Although not always possible, an onsite gym that staff and providers can access to work off the daily stress that comes from working those rough days is a highly valued benefit. Be creative and work within the organization's ability to provide options for employees to engage in stress-releasing activities. Exercise as a de-stressor helps employees' well-being and improves patient satisfaction. Before spending money on a gym benefit, make sure this will be valued by the staff. Consider the age of staff, their interests and time as to whether or not this will be a good benefit to offer.

Other incentives: There are always ways to structure bonus incentives and raises to consider. One of the most appealing incentive options is profit sharing. Such programs give participants a stronger connection and motivation to contribute to the organization's growth. Creative lifestyle incentives such as childcare, pet-sitting, pet insurance and grocery delivery are a few that may be valued.

Each of these options would undoubtedly help maintain morale and promote employment longevity, but no one answer is correct. HR must work with practice leaders to determine what will work best for the employee that will also align with the goals and capability of the practice.

2.3 Improving Workplace Culture through Recognition

What does it mean to improve workplace culture? This discussion explores a proactive approach to cultivating workplace culture advantageously.

According to a report by O.C. Tanner, there are seven powerful best practices to improve workplace culture:[14]

- Building strong employee relationships
- Connecting people to a purpose
- Encouraging frequent employee recognition
- Creating positive employee experiences
- Opening transparency and communication
- Giving teams autonomy they seek
- Scheduling regular and meaningful one-to-ones

The foundation of improving workplace culture is building strong employee relationships that will blossom as the business grows. Leaders play an integral role in shaping workplace culture, and if there is a disconnect between leaders and employees, then the employees are more likely to be disengaged. When employees are disengaged, it can cause problems for any business. Highly engaged employees are imperative to a successful workplace culture that leads to a thriving business.

Leaders need to develop the employees who report to them, and most leaders have a unique opportunity to mentor and advocate for their team. Additional OC Tanner research has shown that when a leader is an active mentor, employees experience:

- 76% increase in feeling part of a larger purpose
- 72% increase in connecting strongly with leaders
- 102% increase in feeling motivated
- 320% increase in favorable perception of the leadership team[15]

Mentorship

A positive, strategic tactic for mentoring is getting to know team members personally. Mentoring employees is a way to help employees grow and advance in their career paths. According to a 2021 Work Institute report, the most common reason employees leave a company is for new career advancement.[16] When leaders view their roles as mentors and practice active listening, employees not only feel heard and seen, but they can also communicate their desire for career advancement. Genuine conversations between leaders and employees make staff feel more appreciated while cultivating a stronger connection to the organization and its purpose. It is vital to remind staff of the organization's purpose. The Work Institute report also says employees are 30% more likely to believe everyone is working towards a common goal when reminders of the organization's purpose are evident in the workplace.

The most impactful facet of improving workplace culture is employee recognition. Recognition is the act of showing appreciation for someone and what they do. Fostering a well-designed, recognition-rich environment increases employee job satisfaction, productivity and morale while decreasing turnover. According to a poll by the Achievers Workforce Institute, 78% of employees said they feel highly engaged when there is strong recognition by the organization of their contribution.[17] People will outperform expectations when they know their work is genuinely appreciated.

Peer Recognition Programs

Several ways to personalize a recognition program for the business are discussed elsewhere in this chapter, but a peer recognition program is sometimes overlooked. Peer-to-peer recognition can be a highly effective tool for improving culture, taking some of the pressure off of leadership to ensure that everyone is given a shot at being recognized. It can be an incredible motivational boost for employees to hear positive feedback about their work from peers.

Positive experiences in the workplace and high employee engagement are directly connected. Understanding the employee experience can lead to improved employee engagement. Remember that the employee experience encompasses every interaction the staff participates in within the organization. The current trend is to take a team approach to facilitate transparency and feedback. Here are a few suggestions on ways to foster good connections through open and diverse communication amongst staff, as well as between leadership and staff:

- Establish a system for employees to voice concerns and offer constructive solutions.
- Prioritize creating regularly scheduled group activities and discussions during work hours.
- Prioritize disseminating communication from the top down to keep staff informed about the business. Commit to distributing communication regularly from senior leadership that is informative, genuinely positive, encouraging and appreciative.

Better communication between staff and leadership allows trust to grow, which invariably leads to more productivity, employee longevity and business growth.

Micromanagement can often be perceived as inefficient, ineffective and antithetical to building trust. A team needs the latitude to set goals, make decisions and manage workloads. Staff is less likely to feel confident and collaborative when not given this option. Employees can thrive working autonomously within set guidelines combined with good guidance and communicated expectations. Autonomy in the workplace is an essential element of employee engagement.

A thriving and contented workplace culture leads to many varied business benefits, including attracting high-caliber staff, retaining staff, good morale, high productivity, continuous process improvement, superior job performance and elevated levels of employee engagement. It is worth investing time to develop, improve and foster the business' workplace culture.

2.4 Optimizing Communication and Culture

Communication means exchanging information, both sending or receiving. Effective communication means listening attentively and conveying information efficiently with empathy. Effective communication is necessary to achieve an organization's goals and is crucial to business success. A Cognisco survey of 400 corporations revealed that poor communication costs an estimated $37 billion annually in lost productivity.[18]

Relationship building plays a pivotal role in communication in the workplace. Maintaining effective communication is foundational to minimizing errors and keeping the team working productively. Effective communication adds to business productivity, cohesiveness among employees and an overall sense of accomplishment. Communication is effective when everyone draws from the same pool of information, leaving little room for misunderstandings or alteration of the message, thus decreasing the potential for conflict.

Exhibit 2.2 Essential Skills Involved with Effective Communication

Active Listening	The first step to establishing effective communication is to be a good listener. Communicating is not just about getting thoughts across and voicing opinions, and it is imperative to remember to listen to comprehend rather than to respond. It is vital to learn not to interrupt others while talking and focus on the speaker to understand their message fully to respond thoughtfully. The Greek philosopher Epictetus said, "We have two ears and one mouth so that we can listen twice as much as we speak."
Body language	Communication is a whole-body discussion, not just the face and brain. When someone is speaking it is essential to be engaged and attentive. Engagement will convey to the speaker that they have been heard and understood. Eye contact with a speaker helps them know the audience is attentive. An occasional nod or smile can encourage a speaker to continue and signal they are being well received.
Effective speech and expression	Tone and volume of voice are essential elements in effective communication to support being clear, concise and conveying confidence. Confidence is vital in getting a point across when expressing thoughts and feelings on an issue, especially to a larger group of people.
Knowing the audience	Speaking to family and friends is usually quite different from talking to colleagues and peers. In the workplace, it is vital to capture the attention of an audience to ensure understanding and compliance, and knowing an audience is imperative to crafting and delivering a message that will be best received.

2.5 Communication Strategies and Tools

Organizations need comprehensive policies for communicating with their employees to ensure employee engagement. Consistent, transparent and clear communication with employees from senior leadership will set the tone for the company—and it must be consistent with the organization's mission, vision and culture.

There are many reasons why effective communication is essential to business success, including:

Exhibit 2.3 Effective Communication Essential to Business Success

Relationships	Trust	Teamwork	Innovation
One of management's primary responsibilities is to encourage effective communication to achieve desired outcomes by ensuring that management and employees are on the same page. The main component of successful relationships is the quality of communication, and a lack of effective communication can make it next to promote productive working relationships in an organization.	Trust-building among the team is essential for effective communication. Listening to different points of view between team members and between management and their teams is vital to building trust that contributes to making good decisions. Effective communication will help foster good working relationships amongst team members as they will trust that everyone is doing their part and fulfilling their responsibilities.	Effective communication helps build a team that will work effectively and efficiently as a unit. An effective team fostered by an environment that encourages open communication will be more engaged and productive. Communication increases employee morale when they feel they can freely express themselves. Effective communication ensures that each team member clearly understands their responsibilities to contribute to the organization's goals.	Effective communication encourages and fosters innovation. When openly brainstorming and sharing ideas are encouraged and enabled, the team can be creative and think freely. The sharing of ideas is essential to business development and growth. Employee morale is also positively impacted, contributing to the organization's overall progress.

Engagement	Accountability	Decision-making	Conflict
According to a recent study by Watson Wyatt Worldwide, engaged employees are twice as likely to be top performers and miss fewer workdays. Effective communication is vital to keep employees motivated and working to meet the organization's goal. When employees feel informed, they work harder and more efficiently. When management effectively communicates with the staff, especially about the value of their work, employees are more satisfied and inspired.	Transparent, effective communication is necessary for employees to know and define expectations. As a by-product of effective communication, a sense of responsibility will increase. The sharing of ideas helps to give each employee purpose and can create a streamlined workflow. When encouraged, collaboration supports the organization's success and fosters a positive work environment where employees enjoy work and perform better.	Effective communication makes it easy to have goal-oriented discussions, and excellent communication invites employees to help determine the purpose and direction of the business.	Effective communication is critical for building strong, cohesive working relationships, which dramatically reduces friction. Any time there is a group of people with different perspectives, conflict can arise. Management must lead by example to create openness to resolve disputes quickly. Senior management, if called upon, needs to be available to give immediate attention to resolving disputes. Nothing will divide a team faster than a conflict ignored and left to fester.

Effective communication can positively affect overall business operations in many ways. In contrast, ineffective communication can be highly detrimental to an organization—increasing the chances for misunderstandings, breaking trust, ruining working relationships and potentially leading to hostility. Leaders and managers need to link communication to the business's goal to develop an effective communication strategy. The goals and objectives of the business need to be considered.

An effective plan includes the elements listed below:

- Top-down communication with senior management setting the tone for all communications and the overall culture
- A budget to allow for the use of various forms of technology
- A process in place to gather feedback for consideration when formatting future messages

- Communication materials and methods that are accessible and easy to understand
- Ensuring every employee has a role in effective communication within the hierarchy of the business
- Managers are responsible for daily contact with the staff and communicating pertinent information, both up and down the chain of command
- Employees are responsible for identifying and voicing concerns and issues, providing constructive feedback to their peers and superiors, and listening effectively

Trust must first be established before expecting honest feedback from employees. When employees are engaged and feel like a valued part of the team, they will offer their opinions. A sure way to ensure failure is to ask employees for feedback then do nothing with the information. This is how to lose employee trust and engagement quickly. Of course, not every suggestion will be brought to fruition as some requests are not possible to implement. But the organization's responsibility is always to acknowledge and, whenever possible, implement change based on employee feedback.

It is essential to listen to staff for what is said and what is not said. Daily observation of operations and employee interactions serve to keep a pulse on what is happening. The "management by walking around" type of observation will create an image of an interested leader who knows what is going on. This style also helps prevent surprise business interruptions from catching management off guard.

How a medical organization's leadership communicates with employees is vital to maintaining the culture. Suggestion boxes sometimes work, but having one-on-one communication is more personal and meaningful. Staff members take more ownership of an issue or suggestion if they feel seen, heard and acknowledged. "Consider a quarterly 'ask me anything' session with different leaders and a cross-section of employees," suggests Cat Graham, founder of Cheer Partners, in a Forbes interview. "Or consider holding 'Friday forums' on the last Friday of each month and choose a topic to review, from wellness benefits employees would like to see or any new program you have rolled out."[19]

Informal one-to-one meetings between employees and their leaders help improve workplace culture. An annual performance appraisal is not the only time for a one-to-one. Remember, to create high employee engagement, it is paramount for the employee to feel heard, seen and valued, so one-to-one sessions are beneficial whenever possible and practical. It is best to strive for open communication in these discussions. Plus, it is good practice to always check with the employee on how they feel in their role, ask if they have suggestions for process improvement and if they need help or guidance with anything. Beyond those standard questions, the optimal value is gained through collaborating with the employee in setting the meeting agenda for an informal discussion.

Effective communication helps individuals get through various tasks of their work-life with ease. When an organization assesses its culture, only then can policies, programs and strategies be established and communicated that support its core purpose and values. The same core values must motivate and unite everyone, from the C-suite to front-line employees.

The quantitative results of more formal surveys and other research can be useful in defining and fostering better culture, to better support business objectives and goals. Here are some strategies for doing so:

- **Develop a cultural assessment instrument:** Many businesses implement an employee survey for this purpose. The survey allows staff to rate the organization on the business culture along with aspects of leadership communication and set expectations.
- **Administer the assessment:** To encourage honesty and eliminate employee fears of retaliation, all employees should take the survey anonymously.
- **Analyze and communicate assessment results:** Leadership can come together and review the survey results, question by question, which will allow them to rate each area of focus on importance.
- **Conduct employee focus groups:** An effective way to communicate survey results to the staff, focus groups also allow for open communication to address any hot survey topics or areas of employee concern.

- **Focus on the question:** Who or what makes us who we are? Leadership must promote and be open to change, consider employee feedback and be willing, when possible, to make changes.

It is important to mention that when leaders use surveys to gather information, employees need to see action from the results. Surveys with no action can result in less satisfied employees and turnover. "What I care about [in surveys] are things that are trending in the organization – what are the things we can say people have a collective feeling about," says Tracy Spears, founder of Exceptional Leader Labs. "When you're not wondering and worrying about what's really going on, you can create loyalty throughout the organization."[20]

With hybrid and remote work becoming increasingly commonplace, promoting and communicating culture can be a challenge. However, it also presents opportunities for HR professionals to focus more on intentionality. Companies can help employees see that their value comes from the role they perform, not their physical location. Researchers from *HBR* suggest three strategies for driving culture and connectedness with hybrid and remote work:[21]

- Shift focus from diffusing culture through the workplace to diffusing it through the work itself.
- Connect through emotional proximity, not physical proximity.
- Shift from optimizing overall culture to fostering microcultures.

Keeping the lines of communication open with the staff through this process is key to success. Assess culture until consensus forms around critical issues. Of course, this depends on employee morale and any uncovered issues. For example, if it is revealed that different units within the business are not working well together, that should become an area of focus.

2.6 Diversity, Equity and Inclusion

Why does recognizing and achieving cultural diversity matter in healthcare? It is easy to get lost in the physical aspects of care delivery and dismiss or ignore the nuances in the quality and sensitivities of delivering care to diverse populations. While the historic COVID-19 pandemic affected everyone, from a patient standpoint, the disease was especially devastating to persons of color and other vulnerable populations.[22] Pandemic events brought to light significant disparities regarding access to quality healthcare, including preventive care, diagnosis and surgery, access to vaccines and access to culturally relevant healthcare information.

The focus on diversity, equity and inclusion (DEI) in the post-COVID era has raised questions and concerns that have become a fundamental norm among a new generation of employees. According to Press Ganey research, 86% of job candidates globally say DEI is important to them. "A diverse and equitable culture is correlated with a strong safety culture, which also impacts patient care solutions," says Dr. Tejal Gandhi, addressing that research. "Healthcare systems must support diversity and equity across the entire employee lifecycle or face even more turbulent years ahead."[23]

By working together as a cohesive unit, healthcare professionals can achieve optimal clinical outcomes. However, there are barriers that providers and staff face as they endeavor to work as a cohesive unit to deliver care due to cultural and social inequities, which can undermine their efforts to operate an effective and inclusive workplace. Issues surrounding gender, socioeconomic status, weight, age, racial and ethnic identity, education or any number of other factors can get in the way of productive work and positive outcomes. These identities or categories of belonging are fundamental to who people are and influence a significant part of how people operate in personal, social, work and other situations.

Overcoming Bias

"Everybody has biases. We literally could not function as humans without them. At any given moment, we are exposed to about 11 million pieces of information, and we can only functionally process about 40 of them. So without biases, we'd be on cognitive overload all of the time," said Jessica Ellis-Wilson, FACMPE, Practical Management and Leadership Consulting. "We have to remember that implicit biases can and often do run counter to what we consciously believe. We can honestly espouse equality and equity for all people and yet still behave in ways that are biased and discriminatory while never even realizing it. We have to identify them within ourselves and then we have to mitigate the effect."[24]

Biases are formed within this concept of self and identity. Bias, by definition, equals preference. Everyone has preferences; bias is simply a reflection of one's preferences. Most people will find that groups with which they associate are culturally similar rather than diverse. By and large, people are biased, or said another way, prefer to associate with people with whom they are similar. Consider how insurability affects how some might view patients, such as if a patient has managed care or Medicaid, and how that might affect how care is delivered. Even private pay patients face bias. Just because someone does not have insurance does not mean they cannot pay for their healthcare services. Often, though, that is the perception. Those perceptions and other biases continue to foster inequity, both in care and in the way employees are treated.

"Our current health system came of age when racial segregation and many other forms of discrimination based on things such as gender identity and sexual orientation, disability and other factors were sanctioned by custom and law," according to the National Health Council. "The U.S. healthcare system has dismantled the outward manifestation of segregated care so that race is no longer the explicit discriminator. However, the legacy system continues to bolster discriminatory practices and has replaced the language of segregation with new discriminators."[25]

Age Discrimination

One area of bias that is often overlooked is age discrimination. According to speaker, author and activist Ashton Applewhite, "It looks like not being invited to meetings. As you get older, it looks like not having training come your way ... not getting opportunities to travel. It looks like being sidelined and then it looks like you are losing your job."[26]

"To be told that the thing that you love to do or that the thing you spent decades getting really good at now renders you useless or renders you without value ... that's crushing," Applewhite continued. "A world of longer lives demands that we work longer, but there is [also] a global labor shortage. So, one solution is [to] hire those hundreds of thousands of older workers who are ready and willing and qualified to work."

As multi-generational workforces are becoming more commonplace, here are some strategies to foster a positive culture and effective communication:

- **Encourage intergenerational collaboration:** Create opportunities for different generations to work together on projects, fostering collaboration, knowledge sharing and mutual learning. Establish mentorship programs where experienced employees can mentor and guide younger colleagues, facilitating the transfer of knowledge and skills.
- **Promote effective communication:** Implement a communication strategy that accommodates the preferences of each generation. Some may prefer face-to-face interactions, while others may prefer digital communication tools like text, email or instant messaging.
- **Provide professional development opportunities:** Offer training and development programs that cater to the diverse learning styles and preferences of different generations. Provide opportunities for continuous learning and skill development, including both traditional and technology-driven platforms.

So what can transform the culture in medical practice organizations to become one of acceptance and inclusion? Communication, again, is the key to understanding; however, there needs to be a safe way to acknowledge differences. It is essential to consider how identities are formed and how socialization influences opinions and outlooks. It is imperative to address the overall environment and interpersonal dynamics from both an internal and external perspective.

- **Look internally:** Assess how socialization, identity and experiences have affected how the practice views its patient community.
- **Look externally:** Consider how patients and staff see the practice and experience the world.
- **Look for commonalities:** between the two points of view and determine if there needs to be a shift.

With this new awareness and information, a practice leader's key challenge is integrating these changes into the practice's culture. Consider the case of a nonprofit organization that provides services to cancer patients' non-medical needs that may fall through the cracks; they implemented training classes around diversity, thinking that providing more inclusive marketing would be sufficient to become a more diverse and equitable organization. Integrating these changes is not only a cultural change, but it takes time and effort to reshape the processes, policies, practices, attitudes and beliefs of the people within the organization to support the change.

After gaining an understanding of these basic concepts, the challenging work of cultural transformation can begin. To begin integrating diversity within an organization's culture, consider some of the following steps:

Exhibit 2.4 Steps for Integrating Diversity into Organizational Culture

Sharpening the lens of awareness

Sharpening the lens of awareness may seem like an easy thing to do, but can be difficult. People typically seek information when they know that an information gap exists.

- Increasing awareness will require consistently assessing interactions with others, especially with those who are different.
- Question the assumptions made about people with whom the practice interacts daily and in casual encounters.
- Consider: are decisions and actions based on facts and objective information, or are they influenced by stereotypes and biases?

Build cultural empathy

Cultural empathy is about communication and respect.

- Listen to understand. The goal is to acknowledge the feelings of others and to consider those feelings regardless of individual experiences. When one's understanding of a person and their culture is limited, be aware and resist finishing sentences an offering advice.
- Avoid generalizing a person's experience based on their culture. Cultural empathy helps to build positive relationship, no matter the differences.

Look for allies and become an ally

Allyship provides an opportunity to educate through a process based on trust and accountability. According to Great Place to Work, "allyship in the workplace means using your personal privilege to support colleagues from historically marginalized communities.

- Allies wield their influence to amplify the voices and elevate the employee experience of their underrepresented coworkers." Everyone fruits of their own success to help pave the way forward.
- Being an ally is about taking small actions that make significant impacts.

Be open to crucial and courageous conversations

Understand that offenses may occur on both sides of an issue.

- There are two sides to every story, and while addressing biases can be scary, living as the object of oppression is hard and scary too.
- Be willing to have open and honest discussions. Ask questions. Listen and speak without judgment. Be open and receptive to feedback.

"Efforts cannot end with creating a workplace comprising people from different backgrounds," according to Compass One Healthcare. "Equity involves making sure healthcare associates have the right tools to effectively do their jobs while ensuring patients have what they need to benefit from the best treatment practices. A diverse staff also helps patients from underrepresented backgrounds to feel more comfortable during their hospital stay. Diversity and inclusion directly affect patient health outcomes and quality of life."[27]

Taking care of individuals in the practice is incredibly important because pushing back against ingrained systems of inequity is challenging work. It is frustrating and tiring, so make sure that time is set aside for personal care and recovery.

Keep the following in mind when dealing with DEI in your practice:

- Know that mistakes will be made and be accountable
- Accept the outcome of mistakes, apologize and rethink what needs to change next time
- Listen to all voices
- Be inclusive with inclusive language
- Be aware and educate the practice on diversity, equity and inclusion

Medical providers are responsible for themselves, their organizations and all the populations they serve. Diversity, equity and inclusion is about the journey and all the experiences along the way, one step at a time.

2.7 Practice in Action

Marie Eslick is Human Resources Director at Apex Dermatology and Skin Center, with 14 locations in Northeastern Ohio. A 12-year-old medical group with more than 200 employees, Apex has focused on providing same-day melanoma treatments in locations with traditionally underserved populations who typically waited six months for care—promoting a more-than-96% cancer survival rate for patients. In addition to general dermatology and medical-grade aesthetics, Eslick says Apex also has a full research facility for medication and procedural trials work.

For Eslick, thinking strategically about HR issues began from her first day on the job. "Before I was brought on, there was no one that had held the position before, so I was basically creating HR from the ground up," she says. "I have free rein and full autonomy to put together a true HR experience. The culture here is people first, and that really means our own people. If we look at the people who are assisting the patients and give them all the tools, supplies, engagement and recognition that they need, they're going to carry that over to the patient experience. The employee experience is paramount for us."

One of Eslick's first projects was launching a formal employee recognition program. "In the past, people might be recognized with a gift card here and there or just an 'attaboy' kind of thing. But I went out and found a platform to use. It's designed to be the area where people can not only put in the accolades, but also everyone would see it. It's been an excellent addition to what we have."

Eslick says Apex has also chosen to articulate its values and mission by sponsoring various charity events throughout the year. They have paid for employee entries to the Miles for Melanoma 5K runs and walks, a national fundraiser for the Melanoma Research Foundation.

To help improve employee communication, Eslick has used a semi-monthly newsletter which focuses on key initiatives and upcoming events, but also covers company policies. "We cover the vision and values, the Apex style of what we value and how it should be utilized daily," she says. "Our founder and owner, Dr. Jorge Garcia-Zuagaga, also sends something out every other week, with his thoughts on what's been going on and how he sees things with Apex. We are a very communicative bunch. From the top down, that communication piece is key."

All Apex employees have a company email account, which helps with the distribution of the newsletters and company updates. Eslick says a more contemporary twist is the use of TeamSpeak, a voice communication and chat system more typically found in the online gaming world. Apex utilizes that platform to again share its vision and values with team members, as well as those who have been honored for superior service. "People can see the feed, and we definitely say which value that person is being recognized for and what they did, how they went above and beyond and why they're receiving the accolades. The feed is huge for us, as well."

Those communication efforts, she explains, have produced plenty of active and positive feedback from even her far-flung staff. "When I go to some of the different clinics, I do hear people comment—'hey, I saw that this happened and that so-and-so was recognized, that's pretty cool, I'm happy to be part of that.' They're talking, they're seeing that employee recognition is a thing and they're engaging. You always want to see that people are engaging. I do see it and I feel it because I hear it."

2.8 Summary

The Great Resignation has been a strong reminder of the value of workplace culture. When employees feel valued and feel that they have an opportunity to grow, they are more likely to stick with their jobs. Improving communication and offering an appropriate range of rewards and benefits are all indications of a positive culture, as are efforts to promote more inclusive behavior and work environments.

To summarize, here are some of the key points discussed in this chapter:

- An organization's culture is defined by the expectations, values and practices it instills into all employees—organizational culture develops best when everyone shares similar expectations.
- Improving workplace culture through mentoring, employee recognition and optimized communication can help maximize a practice's success.
- Incorporating diversity, equity and inclusion into organizational culture can help medical practices work as a cohesive unit to not only fight bias and discrimination, but also to achieve optimal clinical outcomes.
- Effective communication strategies and tools are vital to maintaining a strong organizational culture.

The next chapter will look at more strategic approaches to shaping the operational environment, and the ways that systems and procedures can help improve business outcomes.

Notes

1. AMA. https://www.ama-assn.org/practice-management/private-practices/how -create-vibrant-culture-your-private-practice

2. Press Ganey. https://info.pressganey.com/press-ganey-blog-healthcare-experience -insights/healthcare-employee-engagement-and-outcomes-3-ways-to-shift-from -a-vicious-cycle-to-a-virtuous-cycle

3. Gallup. https://www.gallup.com/workplace/468233/employee-engagement -needs-rebound-2023.aspx

4. HR Cloud. https://www.hrcloud.com/blog/8-employee-engagement-statistics-you -need-to-know-in-2021

5. *Corporate Culture and Performance*, John P. Kotter and James Heskett

6. Great Place To Work. https://www.greatplacetowork.com/certified-company/7011008

7. ianacare. https://ianacare.com/resource-center/elevance-health-case-study/

8. MGMA. https://www.mgma.com/articles/factors-of-a-positive-culture

9. MGMA. https://www.mgma.com/articles/formalizing-values-review-an-organizational -strategy-to-shape-culture

10. MGMA. https://www.mgma.com/articles/living-it-creating-and-maintaining -exceptional-organizational-culture

11. Achievers. https://www.achievers.com/blog/organizational-culture-definition/

12. Great Place to Work. https://www.greatplacetowork.com/resources/blog/creating -a-culture-of-recognition

13. SHRM. https://www.shrm.org/hr-today/news/hr-magazine/0418/pages/how-to -design-a-21st-century-time-off-program.aspx

14. OC Tanner. https://www.octanner.com/global-culture-report

15. OC Tanner. https://www.octanner.com/global-culture-report/2019-leadership

16. Work Institute. https://workinstitute.com/retention-reports/

17. Achievers. https://www.achievers.com/press/achievers-report-uncovers-how -employers-can-drive-retention-amid-the-great-resignation/

18. LinkedIn. https://www.linkedin.com/pulse/cost-ineffective-communication -kelly-waltman/

19. Forbes. https://www.forbes.com/sites/forbeshumanresourcescouncil/2021/01/19 /five-ways-hr-leaders-can-drive-effective-communications-with-employees/?sh =68561eb115f8

20. MGMA. https://www.mgma.com/articles/hitting-the-culture-reset-button-for -your-medical-practice

21. HBR. https://hbr.org/2022/11/revitalizing-culture-in-the-world-of-hybrid-work

22. Harvard Health. https://www.health.harvard.edu/blog/communities-of-color -devastated-by-covid-19-shifting-the-nar rative-2020102221201

23. Press Ganey. https://info.pressganey.com/press-ganey-blog-healthcare-experience -insights/why-healthcare-diversity-and-equity-are-central-to-employee-retention

24. MGMA Insights. https://www.mgma.com/podcasts/leadership-strategies-for -confronting-our-implicit-biases

25. National Health Council. https://nationalhealthcouncil.org/issue/health-equity/

26. MGMA Insights. https://www.mgma.com/podcasts/addressing-ageism-in-the -workplace-with-more-inclusive-policies

27. Compass One Healthcare. https://www.compassonehealthcare.com/blog/diversity -and-inclusion-best-practices-healthcare/

Chapter 3

Employment Lifecycle and Job Analysis

3.1 The Employment Lifecycle Within the Context of Business Strategy

In the United States, hospitals and health systems have been facing persistent staff shortages that became more pronounced in the wake of the COVID-19 pandemic. "The total supply of RNs decreased by more than 100,000 in one year (2021)—a far greater drop than ever observed over the past four decades," according to data from *Health Affairs*, a leading journal of health policy thought and research.[1] Additionally, the United States faces a projected shortage of between 37,800 and 124,000 physicians by 2034.[2] The AMA cites emotional and physical stress and burnout, barriers to care delivery and administrative burdens as factors contributing to the ongoing physician shortage.

But staffing shortages are not relegated to the clinical side of healthcare. The effects of the Great Resignation in recent years are still being felt at multiple positions, as revealed in the *2023 MGMA DataDive Practice Operations* report:[3]

- Front office support staff had a 40% turnover rate in the single specialty aggregate of primary care, nonsurgical and surgical single specialty practice data.

- Single specialty aggregate data put turnover for business operations support staff at 33.3% in 2022.

Given those disruptions, this chapter will look at ways to help develop healthcare employees from the earliest stages of recruitment by giving them the skills and opportunities that help build life-long workers— whether that is with your practice or others in the healthcare field. This chapter will focus on building a strategic human resources management approach while defining the technical aspects of organizing principles, well-defined roles, responsibilities and job descriptions to better guide employees from day one to retirement.

Strategic HR is equal parts organizational and employee focus, which makes the function dynamic and rewarding. Finding win-win solutions that are simultaneously positive for the medical practice and its employees can be highly gratifying, like solving a complex puzzle. If strategic planning offers a framework for business strategy, the employee lifecycle offers a similar roadmap for building a medical group for employees to thrive.

The Employee Lifecycle

The employee lifecycle model, which analyzes the path for workers from pre-employment to separation, includes <u>seven stages</u> of an employee's tenure with an organization. Each stage offers the opportunity to engage employees and to demonstrate how the organization handles people leadership differently than other employers. "When you understand how the employee lifecycle model applies to your organization, it's easier to make informed decisions that will benefit your employees and the organization," explains the Academy to Innovate HR.[4] "Monitoring the different stages of the employee lifecycle will ensure that you can offer great experiences to all employees before, during and after their stay with your company."

Improving the employee lifecycle and the overall experience of your workers can also considerably help reduce employee turnover. This starts even before an employee has begun their job; according to the Brandon Hall Group, strengthening the onboarding stage of the employee lifecycle can help improve new hire retention by 82%.[5]

Exhibit 3.1 Seven Stages of the Employee Lifecycle

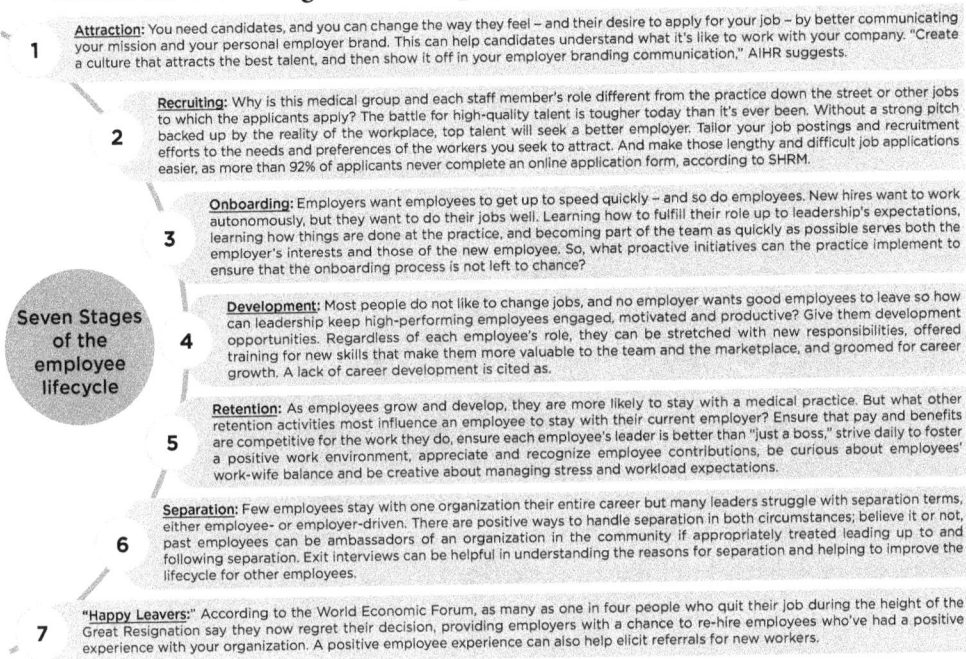

1 **Attraction:** You need candidates, and you can change the way they feel – and their desire to apply for your job – by better communicating your mission and your personal employer brand. This can help candidates understand what it's like to work with your company. "Create a culture that attracts the best talent, and then show it off in your employer branding communication," AIHR suggests.

2 **Recruiting:** Why is this medical group and each staff member's role different from the practice down the street or other jobs to which the applicants apply? The battle for high-quality talent is tougher today than it's ever been. Without a strong pitch backed up by the reality of the workplace, top talent will seek a better employer. Tailor your job postings and recruitment efforts to the needs and preferences of the workers you seek to attract. And make those lengthy and difficult job applications easier, as more than 92% of applicants never complete an online application form, according to SHRM.

3 **Onboarding:** Employers want employees to get up to speed quickly – and so do employees. New hires want to work autonomously, but they want to do their jobs well. Learning how to fulfill their role up to leadership's expectations, learning how things are done at the practice, and becoming part of the team as quickly as possible serves both the employer's interests and those of the new employee. So, what proactive initiatives can the practice implement to ensure that the onboarding process is not left to chance?

Seven Stages of the employee lifecycle

4 **Development:** Most people do not like to change jobs, and no employer wants good employees to leave so how can leadership keep high-performing employees engaged, motivated and productive? Give them development opportunities. Regardless of each employee's role, they can be stretched with new responsibilities, offered training for new skills that make them more valuable to the team and the marketplace, and groomed for career growth. A lack of career development is cited as.

5 **Retention:** As employees grow and develop, they are more likely to stay with a medical practice. But what other retention activities most influence an employee to stay with their current employer? Ensure that pay and benefits are competitive for the work they do, ensure each employee's leader is better than "just a boss," strive daily to foster a positive work environment, appreciate and recognize employee contributions, be curious about employees' work-wife balance and be creative about managing stress and workload expectations.

6 **Separation:** Few employees stay with one organization their entire career but many leaders struggle with separation terms, either employee- or employer-driven. There are positive ways to handle separation in both circumstances; believe it or not, past employees can be ambassadors of an organization in the community if appropriately treated leading up to and following separation. Exit interviews can be helpful in understanding the reasons for separation and helping to improve the lifecycle for other employees.

7 **"Happy Leavers:"** According to the World Economic Forum, as many as one in four people who quit their job during the height of the Great Resignation say they now regret their decision, providing employers with a chance to re-hire employees who've had a positive experience with your organization. A positive employee experience can also help elicit referrals for new workers.

By understanding that employment is a multifaceted journey, HR professionals can bring more value to the working experience and better focus resources across the entire employee lifecycle.

3.2 Employee Value Proposition

As HR formulates the organization's approach to each stage of the employee lifecycle in a way that is sustainable for a medical practice, the final examination of those approaches should be through the lens of a prospective employee. What words should be used when HR summarizes how its organization conducts itself for prospective employees? A way to discuss this is to describe the value an employee receives from working at the practice, or the employee value proposition.

SHRM describes an employee value proposition as "a part of an employer's strategy that represents everything of value that the employer has to offer its employees. Items such as pay, benefits and career development are common, but employers also highlight offerings that are currently in demand—like technology, remote work and flexible scheduling."[6]

The benefits of a well-articulated employee value proposition include:

- Aligning personal values in a more emotional contract between employee and employer
- An increasing commitment of employees to enhance their engagement
- Increasing employee referrals
- Improving the practice's brand appeal
- Building a competitive advantage over other medical practices that is hard to replicate, resulting in improved patient attraction and retention, and thus higher earnings

To better understand the value proposition, frame an employee's view of the practice using these five criteria:

1. Opportunities on the job
2. The financial reward received for doing the job
3. The work done daily
4. The people with whom they work
5. The practice within which they operate

These five benchmarks exist in some balance with each employee, which is a different balance for each. The degree to which HR can uncover how its employees weigh that balance, the better it will be at creating optimal value for employment with the medical practice.

An employee might strongly value only two or three elements of the criteria, but in non-stereotypical ways, that could cause a significant misalignment between them and the practice. Typically, employees desire the highest compensation or total rewards package, with opportunities for growth in their current organization and, more so today, flexibility in their work schedules. If the medical group assumes those are the three core value elements to focus solely on, then be prepared to sacrifice elements of organizational camaraderie and team effectiveness.

A Focus on Culture

According to a study by the Boston Consulting Group, companies that focus on culture were five times more likely to achieve strong results, especially in the ongoing realm of digital transformation, than their competitors.[7] "An adaptive culture provides a foundation for transformation," explains the MIT Sloan Management Review. "Leaders also need to understand that culture is dynamic and that change will happen in their organization, even if they do nothing to guide it."

Many managers have been in a group (or at least are familiar with groups) where there is tension, conflict or even outright fighting between staff members. The repercussions of that environment are clear. Bad patient interactions, worse staff morale and untenable work arrangements mean immediate actions must be taken to minimally correct inappropriate staff behavior or terminate certain team members for destructive team behavior. But can these situations be remedied before they even occur by examining the balance of value provided to employees?

According to AIHR, the use of pre-selection tools such as cognitive testing or a realistic job preview can help offer a picture of both the enjoyable and interesting aspects of a role but also the challenges faced, which helps align expectations between employer and employee while leading to hires who are a stronger fit.[8]

Exhibit 3.2 The Seven Stages of the Selection Process

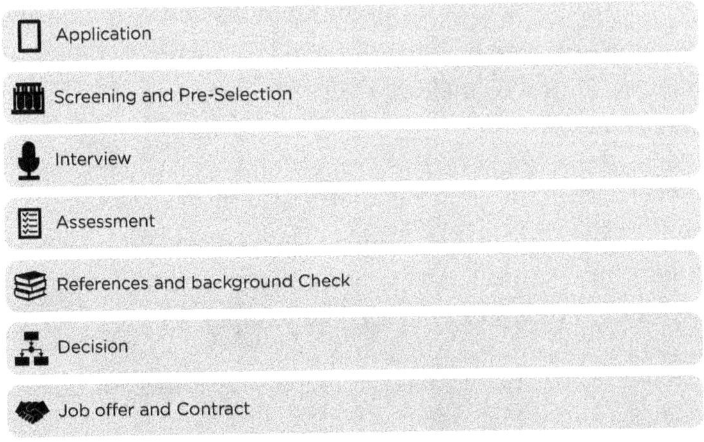

- Application
- Screening and Pre-Selection
- Interview
- Assessment
- References and background Check
- Decision
- Job offer and Contract

If employee selection in the hiring process puts equal emphasis on each element, then answers to behavioral interviewing about the importance and adherence to organizational culture and teamwork become equally as important to pay and opportunities.

If candidates' questions about their work environments deal with prompt pay, opportunities to earn more and what the practice does to keep them trained and progressing through their careers, then it can be an indication that these will be the core values of the new staff member if hired.

If another candidate asks questions about who they'll be working with, how they could create a mentor relationship at the practice or what the group does together for fun during and after hours, it can point to where their values lie.

Therefore, employers need to clearly articulate for each employee, new or long-tenured, how their medical group balances each element of the value proposition to deliver the most value for the medical group. Showing employees what the medical group needs from employees to be successful can be a win-win and eye-opening conversation between employer and employee. Transparently discussing how patient visits earn medical revenue, which in turn pays for staff salaries, explains why showing up on time for a shift or rooming a patient quickly means success for the practice and pay for the employee. Showing a new hire a picture of the end-to-end patient visit experience and all the handoffs between different staff members is an easier way to describe why good teamwork and positive staff relationships are critical to making the work of the group not only efficient but more enjoyable.

Each element of the employee value proposition has a coinciding employer value. For the strategic HR leader, clearly articulating each of those employer benefits is critical. And communicating those benefits to other leaders and staff at the right time is equally important.

Potential activities to further engage employees and gain buy-in include:

- **Identification and recognition**. During the strategic planning process and quarterly review, identify areas where the group is performing well or not in delivering the expected value elements; this recognition can help steer the next quarter's improvement or celebration focus.
- **The Power of Huddles**. Daily or weekly team huddles can be points of reinforcement or recognition about how the group is experiencing a strong realization of employee value and a discussion of how that benefits the group and its patients.

According to Indeed, motivational team huddles from management to individual department levels can align tasks and projects, create actionable plans, build work relationships and assess current progress.[9]

3.3 Systems and Policies to Maximize Employee Value Proposition

Non-healthcare companies such as Amazon and Uber have revolutionized technology and artificial intelligence, proving that once-traditional tangible assets provide a less competitive edge. Likewise, large and small businesses in healthcare should consider a deeper focus on the intangible assets at their disposal. HR provides leadership concerning the most significant intangible asset: its employees. In the "high-touch" business of a medical practice, its people are the differentiator.

Employee engagement, which is discussed at length in later chapters, continues to be a challenge. Many organizations rarely meet their staff's basic needs at various points along the employee lifecycle, and some only turn to HR for a problematic employee issue or when someone unexpectedly gives notice.

In contrast, fostering a strong company culture requires leadership to partner with HR in attracting, acquiring and retaining the best employees. "Leaders play an indispensable role in shaping the culture through values, in adoption and in action," according to an MGMA.com article on shaping culture. "Understanding and appreciating the behavioral implications of leadership actions on culture are instrumental in shaping the future.

Culture is not static and continues to evolve over years and decades, while the foundational values remain intact."[10]

Here are a few things that management can do to help HR get the best out of the staff:

- **Raise expectations for results:** Organizational and people strategies should merge if the practice's employees are its best asset, and the plan is to invest in them. HR needs to be included in making company decisions and share accountability to help the company achieve its goals.
- **Make data-driven decisions:** HR collects employee feedback and performance data, but management needs clear parameters to use the data effectively. Leaders need to work with HR to establish the metrics used for performance appraisals and concur on interpreting feedback.
- **Developing managers:** Managers are often at the center of successful and failed employee relations. According to a Gallup survey, managers account for 70% of the variance in team engagement.[11] Educating and training managers to be more effective is essential since they are primarily responsible for day-to-day staff engagement.

In order to help better facilitate employee engagement and ensure that standards and practices are followed, healthcare practices also need business systems, processes and procedures that help people work together toward the same goal.

Business Systems

A system is a set of processes, tools and people that work together toward the same goal. Meanwhile a process is typically documented for the business and used as a reference. According to the American Academy of Family Physicians, the practices and procedures of business systems such as scheduling systems, digital appointment confirmations and other electronic tools can also help create a 20% increase in net income for a small healthcare business when used correctly.[12] Systems processes in the industry bring separate work teams together.

These systems help to make a business maintain and grow, as well as improving patient satisfaction, simplifying the time-consuming process of appointment scheduling and simplifying both documentation and billing.[13] A systematic, standardized approach to building an organization eliminates guesswork. It tells employees exactly how to accomplish tasks or jobs. Employees may come and go, but the effective business system stays the same.

As Otis Lewis, MHA, CHFP, FACMPE, writes, "The outcomes or expectations of a task should not be subject to the person who is completing it. Unintended outcomes are three times more likely when standardization processes are not followed."[14] An effective business system aims to give proper education and opportunities to all employees. This training method ensures the efficiency and effectiveness of every process. Effective business systems help to increase employee engagement as everything is clearly defined. Bringing on new employees is also simplified; there is no question about expectations or responsibilities. It is a checklist of standard operating procedures for employees. Therefore, the systems run as a process and keep the teamwork approach in all aspects of the job.

Creating the appropriate systems for an organization can take much work and thought, but is well worth the effort. Here are some variables to consider:

- Who will do a particular task?
- How does management want the job completed?
- When do they need to do it?

Process Alignment

Work collaboratively with the practice's team to create the best method for processes. Once agreed upon, put it in writing as the best practice to achieve the organization's goal. Make the documented process easy to follow, outlining each step and leaving nothing for interpretation. The process becomes an educational tool and a resource for later reference. This process can then become a standard operating procedure (SOP). The key to process implementation is to follow the sequential steps as written. Over time, the process will become second nature. Remember that it is essential to schedule process reviews over time with the mindset that consistent process reviews will improve efficiency. It is necessary to revisit processes to streamline procedures for a growing business. Regular inspection will help to ensure employee engagement and end-users often recommend the most beneficial changes to operations.

Policies and Procedures

Formalizing HR policies and procedures is essential, even for a small practice. HR policies are formal rules and guidelines put in place to manage employees. "HR policies provide employees with a framework to understand the advantages derived from the processes' consistency," explains Loop Health. "The policies help a company exhibit, externally and internally, that it meets the needs for diversity, ethics and training, along with commitment regarding corporate governance and rules."[15] Without clear, concise, transparent guidelines to be followed, misunderstandings are inevitable. Building trust between employees and employers is vital for success, and clear policies are needed to be effective. Setting clear ground rules helps ensure that everyone stays on the same page. HR procedures are step-by-step instructions for actions to ensure compliance with HR policies. A core function of human resources management is defining policies and procedures.

HR procedures often evolve into SOP documents for the practice. These documents often become necessary resource materials referred to by the staff and used in new hire orientation. Many areas of human resource management are covered and outlined by HR policies such as:

- Recruitment
- Dress code
- Paid and unpaid time off
- Employee evaluation
- Termination

HR policies aim to protect a business from legal claims, but equally important is to foster a culture of trust, fairness and inclusion. Here are some reasons why it is crucial to establish HR policies and publish them for the staff:

- Protection from legal claims filed against the practice
- Communicate the conditions of employment
- Set employee expectations
- Help address employee grievances and disputes
- Can expedite decision-making on HR issues
- Create a healthy work environment
- Ensure equality and fairness

When writing effective policies, it is essential to decide upon a format and be consistent. For instance, all policies should be easily accessible by the staff and stored in a shared drive or company intranet where they can regularly access them. Best practice recommends that all the business policies are in the employee handbook and posted on a company intranet or shared drive. Each policy should include the following:

- Policy name and title
- The effective date (to be clear when to begin enforcing the policy)
- Policy writer (the person/department for answering questions about said policy)
- Purpose of the policy
- Scope and applicability (to whom or which department the policy applies)

As the workplace evolves and the business grows, keep updating and/or revising policies as applicable. Employees really do look to policies for guidance on assorted topics, such as use of new technology. The social media revolution has considerably affected workplace relationships and created privacy nightmares that pose significant risks to a practice, including reputational risk, employment law risk, morale risk and regulatory risk. In this era, social media policies must be part of every employee handbook. There is no exact list of policies that apply to every healthcare business, but several are considered critical to any organization.

Employees can typically find the following standard policies in their organization:

Exhibit 3.3 Standard Policies and Procedures

Code of conduct: establishes acceptable employee behavior, dress code, punctuality, harassment in the workplace and alcohol/drug use.	**Recruitment:** outlines criteria for new hire selection and the onboarding process.	**Termination:** outlines the amount of notice required for separation and how resignations are submitted.
Working hours: outlines employee work schedules and whether set hours are flexible and addresses overtime.	**Attendance:** addresses how many absences are allowed before employee discipline is initiated, outlines proper procedures for employee absence notification and who must be notified.	**Performance evaluation:** outlines the job performance evaluation process, indicates which metrics are measured and whether performance measures merit a pay increase. Evaluations are often a great motivational tool for staff
Health and Safety: regardless of the work environment, accidents happen. This policy outlines how employees are to behave and perform duties to ensure a safe workplace.	**Expense reimbursement:** outlines what the company will reimburse, how to submit expense reports to the company and when to expect funds.	**Benefits and compensation:** outlines pay periods, payment frequency and employer benefits such as 401k, medical, dental, vision and life insurance.
	Paid leave: indicates the number of paid days off, sick time and company holidays allocated yearly, how much vacation time an employee can take at once, and how to request paid time off.	

Sexual misconduct, harassment or unsafe work practices occurring in the workplace may cause a company to write new or revise policies to address the problem. Depending on the circumstances it is essential to deliver education or otherwise inform employees of the new policy to minimize the likelihood of recurrence.

Healthcare employers also have special risk issues related to the HIPAA Privacy Rule, which dictates social media in the healthcare workplace. Misuse of social media or use of smartphone cameras in the practice can result in HIPAA violations due to mishandling of sensitive patient information. Medical practices should have written social media policies regarding both online activity by employees and potential employer monitoring. The policy should clearly state an employee's expectation of privacy (or lack thereof) while engaging in social media at work with medical practice computers, networks and equipment, along with the extent to which the employer monitors such activities. This policy should be reviewed and updated regularly.[16]

Another way to view human resources is to think of it as the employee relations department. HR should be the one-stop shop for employees. HR is where employees get clarification on published policies, ask benefit questions, express training needs and seek guidance. It is vital to ensure that HR policies align with business objectives as well as federal, state and local laws, some of which will be discussed in Chapter 7.

Strategic human resource management is defined as merging business strategy with HR practices to achieve the organization's overall goal. The premise is that companies must integrate their HR practices within the scope of overall business objectives, which ensures that the business strategy and objectives align with the HR practices and policies. The business world has changed, and HR management has become viewed as promoting and supporting the organization's business objectives— not just a department responsible for helping manage employees. It has become imperative for companies to take a "people first" approach in administering their HR practices to maintain sustainable business growth. Considering this, the role of HR is called upon to be hands-on and proactive. A proactive method needs to be the priority of both management and HR when dealing with employees. This HR methodology encompasses hiring, onboarding, policy creation, training, evaluations and other areas as needed. An organization's success hinges on the people who affect operations the most. HR and management must have a cohesive relationship.

Getting the best from employees and the business is a team effort. HR protects employers and employees by enforcing policies and procedures, and these policies help keep everyone aware of the rules and regulations in place. The success of HR departments directly affects the organization's success, serving as the backbone supporting consistent processes, effective systems and an optimum work environment.

3.4 Organizational Design – Aligning Staff Needs with Business Outcomes

As Human Resource Management is appropriately incorporated into the strategic direction of the medical practice, the strategic HR leader must then lead a conversation about how best to arrange the roles within an organization to get the most return from its investment in human capital. "Human capital is the economic value of the human being in a market economy, in terms of both personal income accrual and organizational productivity," says Angelo Scozia, of Willis North America, an employee benefits and insurance brokerage company. "Enterprises evaluate a person in terms of return on investment in both the short and long terms. Initial investment is through compensation and benefits, which pays for the best human capital investment inputs and, if done right, retains these people for the long term."[17]

Unfortunately, for many practices, a decision to cut the number and type of staff can have an adverse effect on operational success, even though staff salaries and benefits represent the largest single cost they face. "All you need is the right people doing the right things and your problem is solved, right?" says David N. Gans, MSHA, FACMPE, "Unfortunately, staffing realities are much more complex, and there is strong evidence to suggest that most practices exercise false economy in staffing. In other words, they reduce the number of staff to the point that production is constrained and overall profitability is reduced."[18]

Business and HR leaders should discuss in depth and in great detail the types of roles the organization needs to best deliver care to their communities. Unless a new practice is starting, there is a current organizational model with which operations are executed by today. But an analysis of the effectiveness of that organizational model can lead to improvement opportunities or resource scaling that the current model might not deliver. There is no single, "correct" organizational model for a medical group;

there are a handful of models that, depending on the organizations' scale and scope, might be a good fit.

Consideration for new or modified organizational structures might include:

- Changes in economic conditions
- New types of patient care
- Different employee roles
- Collaborative systems for allocating resources and sharing authority

When leadership, led by HR, discusses and agrees on potential changes to organizational structures, the involvement of downline staff in the change is imperative for improved buy-in and ultimate success of the new structure. Task forces and committees can help managers smooth the way for structural change by stimulating participation and improving coordination. These staff members or teams aren't given the opportunity to veto a leadership decision but should be involved in optimizing the processes around the new structure, so it achieves the desired outcomes.

Organizations that are reorganizing need to take coordination to a higher level. Having separate and independent silos is not effective or sustainable. A reorganization is a good time to integrate finance and marketing, administrative and clinical, physicians and support staff, the board of directors and the senior management team. According to *Physicians Practice*, this also calls for creating and defining an organizational chart that outlines the division of work, the line and flow of authority, the span of control, as well as delegation, decentralization and departmentalization.[19] Coordinating each department's plans and activities can vastly improve the chances for developing a structure that only fits planned changes but allows the medical practice to thrive.

It is the role of a strategic HR partner to work collaboratively with each function to define the job responsibilities of each role within the function. Specifically, a strategic HR partner should be asking pointed questions about job functions that are changing, being added, or being removed to better understand how each role is changing and staying the same. These points of clarification then lead into discussions about the reliance between roles inside and outside the function. With a clear understanding of each role's fit with others in the organization, reporting structures can be formed around individual and joint accountabilities.

For example, a medical practice has decided to add patient financial counselors to its team. The added cost of bringing on staff has been justified by the amount of revenue those positions will capture instead of going to bad debt. But there is a question of whether the roles should report into the accounting and finance function or the operations team, who manages the front desk and clinic workflow. Both teams can make compelling cases that the role's job responsibilities fit with either function. So an analysis of the role's key processes—such as patient communication, payment policy education, patient financial planning, processing payments and patient handoffs with other team members—make it clear to the organization that while the role has a tie to finance, the role will report into the operations function because the key processes it performs intersects mainly with those staff members—front desk, scheduling, and medical assistants—far more than finance, even though the role's responsibilities are to improve the financial performance of the organization.

3.5 Job Analysis

Analyzing the jobs in a medical practice supports managing HR responsibilities and helps managers and employees to understand the nature of the practice's work. According to the U.S. Office of Personnel Management (OPM), "job analysis is the foundation for all assessment and selection decisions."[20] A job analysis can accomplish various objectives, including the why, the how or the need for a position. It can also provide a source of legal defensibility of assessment and selection procedures, the OPM adds. Redefining functions might happen for multiple reasons in any area of the medical practice. A job analysis should be done at least annually or for every position vacancy.

Job analysis helps everyone gain a better understanding of the extent of an individual's work, the relationship of the work to the practice and the qualifications the individual must have to fulfill all of the job tasks.

Analyzing all of the jobs in the practice assists in managing HR responsibilities, and helps managers and employees understand more fully the nature of the practice's work.[21]

A job analysis consists of three major components:

- Evaluation of tasks and competencies
- Subject matter rating of the duties and competencies
- Identify tasks or competencies to be eliminated or reassigned

The parameters for employee skills assessed in a job analysis include essential functions and related duties, the occupation involved, supervisor and nonsupervisory responsibilities, physical demands, work conditions and technology requirements. It should also identify the necessary knowledge, skills and abilities, as well as performance standards. The requirements for job analysis include three elements:

Exhibit 3.4 Three Elements of a Job Analysis

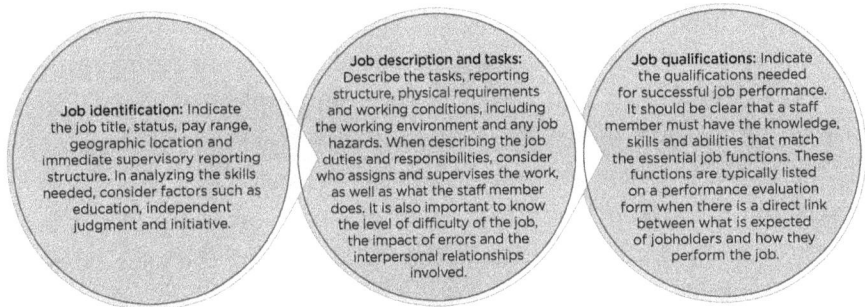

Job identification: Indicate the job title, status, pay range, geographic location and immediate supervisory reporting structure. In analyzing the skills needed, consider factors such as education, independent judgment and initiative.

Job description and tasks: Describe the tasks, reporting structure, physical requirements and working conditions, including the working environment and any job hazards. When describing the job duties and responsibilities, consider who assigns and supervises the work, as well as what the staff member does. It is also important to know the level of difficulty of the job, the impact of errors and the interpersonal relationships involved.

Job qualifications: Indicate the qualifications needed for successful job performance. It should be clear that a staff member must have the knowledge, skills and abilities that match the essential job functions. These functions are typically listed on a performance evaluation form when there is a direct link between what is expected of jobholders and how they perform the job.

Role clarity is the base for job analysis; it is essential when filling vacancies to define the role of a job for a possible new hire or determine if a position is still needed or when creating a new job to accommodate new requirements of the business, or to react to pressures or new regulations, as occurred frequently during the COVID-19 epidemic. A 2022 MGMA *Stat* poll found that more than 58% of medical groups reported updating job descriptions or duties in the past year to help improve staff recruitment. Owing to the challenges related to recruitment in recent years, the most commonly updated job descriptions included medical assistants, remote and hybrid positions, along with front desk, patient contact and care coordination positions.[22]

There are many elements to address when analyzing a position. Methods for job analysis include questionnaires, interviews, checklists, diaries, observations, activity samplings and critical incidents. Talking to managers, customers and experts can help analyze. Reexamining documents like planning portfolios and reports of accomplishments can help managers and HR departments re-establish a criterion for a job description. It is essential to examine future-focused documents such as a strategic plan. These documents can predict the future of the practice or policy paperwork. It's important to talk to senior leaders and policymakers to help shape future policies to meet consumer dynamics. Learning from senior executives, policy analysts and other subject matter experts can help future approaches.

Part of the job analysis process is to ask departing employees or staff their views on how effective the work is in its current state. Exit interviews give a human resources department or employer a better understanding of the job description. The exit interview is the best way to hear firsthand about the reasons that your employees—from physicians to office staff—leave the company. A simple survey can also be sent to those who have left in the last year.[23] This process can also help determine the strength or production of a unit or group of workers. After considering all these factors, the task is to state the job's essential functions clearly.

Predicting likely future job changes or updates is essential when evaluating a job analysis. It may be hard to predict future behaviors of a position but looking at a past blueprint of behavioral changes can help predict this change. Evaluating job changes over the past five years, and evaluating what changed, can help reframe a position. Consider past changes or employees and rethink the approach toward the competencies or tasks for a position to help determine future issues with technology or organizational structure. This approach can also help craft a better organizational structure for future employees working in analyzed positions and help them succeed in the company.

SAMPLE EXIT INTERVIEW QUESTIONS

Exit interviews are valuable opportunities to gather feedback from departing employees, which can help organizations identify areas for improvement and enhance retention efforts. In a healthcare organization, it's important to conduct exit interviews with sensitivity due to the nature of the industry. Exit interviews should be conducted in a confidential and non-confrontational manner, with the primary goal of gathering constructive feedback. Ensure that departing employees feel comfortable expressing their views and that the information collected is used to inform improvements in the organization's practices and culture.

Here are some sample exit interview questions that the HR department can ask departing employees:

1. **General Information**
   - Name (optional):
   - Department/Unit:
   - Job Title:
   - Last Working Day:
   - Reason for Leaving:

2. **Job Satisfaction**
   - What factors contributed to your decision to leave [Organization Name]?
   - Were there any specific aspects of your job that you found particularly rewarding?
   - Were there any aspects of your job that you found challenging or frustrating?

3. **Work Environment**
   - How would you describe the work culture and environment at [Organization Name]?
   - Did you feel supported by your colleagues and supervisors during your time here?
   - Were there any workplace issues or concerns that you felt were not adequately addressed?

4. **Supervision and Leadership**
   - How would you rate the quality of supervision you received during your tenure here?
   - Were there any specific instances or concerns related to leadership or management that you would like to share?

5. **Training and Professional Development**
   - Did you feel that you had access to adequate training and professional development opportunities?
   - Were there any skills or knowledge areas where you felt additional training could have been beneficial?

6. **Compensation and Benefits**
   - Were you satisfied with your compensation and benefits package?
   - Did you receive timely and clear information about your benefits and payroll?

7. **Work-Life Balance**
   - How did you perceive the work-life balance at [Organization Name]?
   - Were you able to maintain a healthy work-life balance during your employment?

8. **Suggestions for Improvement**
   - What recommendations do you have for [Organization Name] to enhance the employee experience and retain talent?
   - Are there specific areas where you believe the organization could make positive changes?

9. **Future Career Goals**
   - What are your future career plans or goals after leaving [Organization Name]?
   - Do you have any feedback or suggestions for [Organization Name] on how it can better support employees in their career development?

10. **Overall Experience:** Overall, how would you describe your experience working at [Organization Name]? Is there anything else you would like to share about your time here or your reasons for leaving?

Additional Comments: Is there anything else you would like to add or any comments you believe would be helpful for us to know?

Inspiring
healthcare
excellence.

MGMA

Typically, an in-house human resources professional coordinates the job analysis process, or a consultant who is a specialist in job analysis is hired for just this purpose. It is imperative to document actions, strategies, techniques and activities during the job analysis process. It is wise to plan for delays and setbacks and to anticipate resistance to change when transitioning job duties, which could come from the staff being evaluated and reconfigured. Despite various challenges, the job analysis process is valuable and crucial to establishing or maintaining a cohesively functioning business.

3.6 Roles, Responsibilities & Job Descriptions

The logical output of a robust job analysis are role and responsibility documentation, typically in the form of job descriptions. Job descriptions simply explain the knowledge, skills and attributes (KSAs) that a person needs to complete a defined set of tasks or responsibilities of a job within the organization. But past its formal purpose at the individual level for job clarity and purpose, collectively, job descriptions document ALL of the critical tasks of a medical group and, of course, who should perform them. This collective meaning becomes hugely important when considering the organizing principles of the group.

At an individual level, a job description is a communication vehicle. Hiring is nearly impossible and never successful without a well-crafted job description which forms the job posting, determines the interview questions to vet candidates and becomes the foundation for a new employee's onboarding. A job description is the vehicle to drive ongoing performance management—is the job being done according to a set of expectations, so the practice knows those tasks are being done and done well? The very ability to get work done in a clearly defined way between multiple people inside a medical group is formed by well-articulated job descriptions that delineate who performs what task. The benefits are equally important when taken from the employees' perspective. The employee is looking for a documented set of expectations of what they are to accomplish in the job on a day-to-day basis.

Workforce Planning

The collection of job descriptions offers one more collective benefit to the medical group and employee alike: workforce planning. A large medical practice with more than one site, one consisting of multiple specialties or a group operating as part of a larger medical system, all have workforce needs with scale. The strategic and operational considerations below are all reliant on advance workforce planning conversations and plans that drive a variety of organizational structure considerations:

- How many nurses are needed to fulfill the patient volume for the day or week?
- Can the same front desk staff cover multiple sites if check in processes and technology are different due to a merger or acquisition?
- If a new site is opened, will existing staff be asked to cover at that location until staff dedicated to that location are hired?

The time an organization spends workforce planning entirely depends on the current complexity of the operation or its future need to change. A small group who is adding a service line will need to engage in workforce planning to ensure the success of the new service line. And a large regional, multi-specialty, multi-site organization with a steady workforce will need only minimal time spent in workforce planning.

Staffing Crunch

Even after the height of the COVID-19 pandemic passed, some medical groups couldn't reopen to full capacity due to a lack of staff to see patients. Some 56% of medical groups polled by MGMA in April 2023 said staffing remains their biggest productivity roadblock.[24] Workforce plans contain elements of both environmental factors and internal needs. When external factors are unclear, as is often the case, even greater clarity must be achieved regarding the internal staffing needs. Clarity on what the group must have to operate into the future can help narrow the focus on what is needed from a vague market.

Keep in mind that a new operational philosophy is also emerging that shifts the focus from jobs alone to a skills-based approach, offering more long-term flexibility and longevity for both employees and employers in a changing labor and technological market, according to Deloitte.[25] Jobs have been the traditional structure for work for centuries, but confining work to a set of standardized tasks and then making decisions based on job alone hinders organizational ability, growth and innovation. By decoupling some work from the job, broadening it so it is focused on problems to be solved, outcomes to be achieved or value to be created, employees can be freed from being defined by their jobs and instead be seen as whole individuals with skills and interests that can be deployed to work matching their interests, as well as evolving business priorities and patient needs.

3.7 Organizing Principles

Organizational design principles are applied so a medical group can make decisions at all levels of the practice. Organizational design clarifies hierarchy and authority and determines how information flows around the organization. Most think of a traditional centralized, top-down organizational structure when considering a medical practice's organizing principles. In truth, many organizations run much more decentralized, with stand-alone organizational structures inside one corporate entity.

By definition, organizational structures can be either centralized or decentralized. The typical CEO- or physician-driven leadership mantle, with staff reporting through a variety of reporting lines, to said CEO or physician, is the well-known centralized model. The most decentralized model is that of a private equity venture, which owns or has stake in a variety of groups (large or small) and with some oversight lets them run their operation and make almost every decision large and small without interference. "In the end, this is an individual decision," says Dr. Matthew Zimm, a Pennsylvania ophthalmologist, in talking about his decision to enter a private equity partnership. "It is not for everyone, but trends in the healthcare market suggest that private independent practices are not in the future."[26]

There are multiple examples of organizational structures that operate in the middle, as well. Large integrated delivery systems often match this description, especially during and after a period of acquisition. There exists a centralized hierarchy leading the large medical group, which determines strategy and long-term direction of the group. And day-to-day, a site of care or purchased group will continue to operate without much, if any, oversight from the centralized leadership body. In that example, eventually the de-centralization becomes more centralized, hence many of the conflicts tied to integration that those systems experience in those organizing exercises.

There is no right or wrong organizational principle of centralization or decentralization, nor operating model. However, because centralization within a functional model is the predominant structure of most medical groups, it is within this model more examples of analysis will occur here. Regardless of the operating model, a strategic HR leader must endeavor to explore improvements to the operating structure, even if the overall principles and model don't change. As more groups explore and adopt value-based care, the organizational design of groups has come under scrutiny. With new roles like care coordinators, changed nursing and educator roles and new skills for managed care contracting resources, the corresponding questions about to whom these resources report and who should guide their work have also been discussed at great length.

Every organization handles changes to org structure differently, but best practice is to weigh the costs and benefits of organizing new roles with alternative choices, and getting as many opinions as comfortable before making a decision. Care coordinators likely will sit in a clinical care team managed by a physician or nurse leader. But another option could have them report to a customer contact center with scheduling. As groups add services, merge or acquire other groups and have significant staff turnover as many have, organizational structure should be evaluated to ensure the group is organized to produce the most efficient and effective management of their most expensive investment—their people.

3.8 Practice in Action

Dawn Plested, JD, MBA, FACHE, is a healthcare management consultant with MGMA, based in Atlanta. Plested says a thorough job analysis is necessary to optimize current staffing, and better plan for any fluctuations, as well as serving as a way of establishing your practice's workplace culture. "I very much recommend interviewing your current employees to understand what the job requirements are. Often, we'll put together a job description, but it's pretty far removed from the reality of boots on the ground, day to day. Observe the tasks being performed by your current staff—things that maybe they aren't even thinking of. Collect your data from your employees about their roles, and then break down those job tasks into components and build your job descriptions from there. Have a really strong sense of what your mission, vision and values are as you do that. Who you hire has the biggest determinant of what your culture will actually be like."

When conducting a job analysis and trying to optimize organizational design, Plested says patient load is a key consideration in developing a staffing plan for a medical practice. "You're going to want to consider the number of patients that are being seen daily, and the type of patient—their demographics, their age, their health status, their needs. You also want to look at what the fluctuations are. Are you experiencing a momentary blip in practice or patient volume? I think almost every practice experienced that for a moment during the pandemic—they had extreme surges, and they had times where patient volume was at an ebb. You also want to consider your specialization. Different medical specialties require different skills and staffing configurations, and depending on that, it can be extremely difficult to recruit the needed staff. So you really want to consider that as you onboard people and think about how difficult it will be to replace those individuals. You also want to consider regulatory compliance."

Thinking of the future of a medical practice, Plested says a strategic approach is helpful. "I'm always a fan of strategic planning and long-range thinking. Are there other offerings that can supplement what we're giving our patients, that will help give you a more robust and full-scope care delivery system? You have to think about your financial considerations and what the budget looks like. Can you afford it? Can you not afford it? I think we in healthcare have a way we've always done things, and it's worked. But it's not working these days. So you need to have a little bit of flexibility and a willingness to be adaptable and adjust your staffing accordingly."

That said, Plested reminds HR practitioners that trimming employees to save money also comes with its own risks, especially given the current labor market. "Often when times are tight, staffing is something that gets looked at and cut pretty quickly, and is viewed as a drain on revenue. But if you're running short-staffed, that can cost you revenue. So you have to be pretty thoughtful about that. In the past couple of years there's been a staffing crisis, particularly in certain areas. Hiring MAs and LPNs have been really challenging, but across the spectrum, staffing will continue to be a challenge, with unpredictable patient volumes. But, overworking your staff can be a deadly spiral where you're short-staffed and you're really leaning on your great, hard-working staff, but you're burning them out. It's very hard to replace good staff."

3.9 Summary

Seeing workers for the value and skills they offer—and using job analysis and organizational design to help make better staffing decisions—are all part of a more strategic approach to the broader employee lifecycle. A careful dedication to job descriptions and responsibilities will also help clarify employee roles and help a medical practice create a more compelling employee value proposition.

Key points discussed in this chapter include:

- Each stage the employment lifecycle offers an opportunity to engage employees and to demonstrate how the organization handles people leadership differently than other employers.
- Employers need to clearly articulate for new and tenured staff how their medical group balances each element of the employee value proposition to deliver the most value for the organization.
- Maximizing employee value proposition involves building effective business systems, process alignment as well as policies and procedures.
- It is the role of a strategic HR partner to work collaboratively with each function to define the job responsibilities of each role within the function. Analyzing the jobs in a medical practice supports managing HR responsibilities and

helps managers and employees to understand the nature of the practice's work.

- Organizational design principles allow medical groups to make decisions at all levels of the practice by clarifying hierarchy and authority while determining how information flows around the organization.

The next chapter will examine how competitive compensation and benefits design can also be a compelling factor in attracting and retaining staff.

Notes

1. Health Affairs. https://www.healthaffairs.org/content/forefront/worrisome-drop-number-young-nurses

2. AMA. https://www.ama-assn.org/practice-management/sustainability/doctor-shortages-are-here-and-they-ll-get-worse-if-we-don-t-act

3. https://mgma.com/data-report-practice-operations-2023

4. AIHR. https://www.aihr.com/blog/employee-life-cycle/

5. Brandon Hall Group. https://b2b-assets.glassdoor.com/the-true-cost-of-a-bad-hire.pdf

6. SHRM. https://www.shrm.org/resourcesandtools/tools-and-samples/hr-glossary/pages/employee-value-pr oposition-evp.aspx

7. BCG. https://www.bcg.com/publications/2023/innovation-culture-strategy-that-gets-results

8. AIHR. https://www.aihr.com/blog/selection-process-practical-guide/

9. Indeed. https://www.indeed.com/career-advice/career-development/team-huddle-

10. MGMA. https://www.mgma.com/articles/shaping-a-culture-implications-for-leaders

11. Gallup. https://news.gallup.com/businessjournal/182792/managers-account-variance-employee-engagement.aspx

12. AAFP. https://www.aafp.org/pubs/fpm/issues/1999/0900/p20.html

13. CollaborateMD. https://www.collaboratemd.com/blog/medical-practice-management/

14. MGMA. https://www.mgma.com/articles/enhancing-practice-operations-through-process-standardization

15. Loop Health. https://www.loophealth.com/post/importance-of-hr-policies

16. MGMA. https://www.mgma.com/articles/social-media-and-the-physician-practice-workplace

17. Physicians Practice. https://www.physicianspractice.com/view/value-human -capital-medical-practices

18. MGMA. https://www.mgma.com/articles/cost-efficiency-with-medical-group -staffing

19. *Physicians Practice*. https://www.physicianspractice.com/view/medical-practice -organizational-structure

20. US Office of Personnel Management. https://www.opm.gov/policy-data-oversight /assessment-and-selection/job-analysis/

21. MGMA. *Volume 3: Human Resource Management*. P. 11-13.

22. MGMA. https://mgma.com/mgma-stats/having-trouble-hiring-practice-staff-it -might-be-time-to-update-job-descriptions

23. MGMA. https://www.mgma.com/mgma-stat/finalizing-your-physician-retention -strategies-amid-worsening-shortages

24. MGMA. https://mgma.com/mgma-stats/as-healthcare-staffing-woes-linger -reduced-capacity-remains-the-biggest-roadblock-to-productivity

25. Deloitte. https://www2.deloitte.com/us/en/insights/topics/talent/organizational -skill-based-hiring.html

26. Fierce Healthcare. https://www.fiercehealthcare.com/finance/industry-voices -private-equity-investment-healthcare-making-positive-impact-especially

Chapter 4

Compensation and Benefits Design

4.1 Compensation Structure and Strategy

Competitive pay remains fundamental to attracting and retaining staff, especially during turbulent times. According to the Brookings Institute, median pay among nursing assistants, medical assistants and other healthcare support workers was just $13.48 an hour during the COVID-19 pandemic, despite the increased demands and risks associated with their jobs—leaving many employees feeling "underpaid, undervalued and non-essential."[1] Since then, a systemic change in the American service economy has seen entry-level jobs in food service, hospitality or even delivery companies begin to offer wages and benefits competitive to those in healthcare. Workers have choices, so what will it take for them to continue to make the healthcare industry their priority?

This chapter will address how compensation planning at all levels—from executives and highly-trained salaried employees to part-time workers—must be designed in a competitive fashion. Benefits plan design and administration is more important than ever, with a focus on the right mix of health, wellness and paid-time-off options for all workers.

When determining an organization's compensation structure, its overall business model must be reviewed to ensure alignment. How the organization or the business operates will help guide the comprehensive compensation plan and structure.

For example, a smaller-sized healthcare business that is privately owned and operated may have leeway and flexibility to pay differently than a large-sized practice in which multiple individuals may occupy the same job title. According to Wolters Kluwer, physicians employed in private practice medicine can expect to earn an average of more than $300,000 annually, versus hospital pay of about $278,000 or non-profit pay of about $228,000.[2] Subsequently, the opposite may be true for a larger organization within a network, multi-state or national organization that could have various limitations on what the practice can offer due to rules and policies governing creating like-paying jobs and benefits.

To address this from a strategic standpoint, consider the following questions:

- What is the organization's overall business strategy? The compensation structure must align with the overall business strategy.
- What type of structure would best serve the organization? Does the compensation structure need to be solidified and reviewed annually, or can it be nimble and flexible, given the surrounding location or environment?
- Is the practice a highly structured organization or a more adaptable one?
- Will the information be shared with employees, or is the information solely for leadership or management?
- Will the organization use internal resources to create the compensation program or outsource the project? Many organizations look to outside consultants for assistance or even to create an entire program.

Once answers to these questions are crystallized, and there is clarity around how the compensation strategy should be approached, the next step is to design the compensation program.

Completing a wage and benefits survey in surrounding areas is advisable before designing a compensation plan in competitive marketplaces. It is also advantageous to complete a survey annually or as often as needed based on changes to the local financial and market landscape.

Emerging from the post-pandemic era has vastly accelerated the number of vacancies, as workers facing burnout, low job satisfaction, and hybrid or remote work environments have sought employment in other industries or with more work flexibility. That has affected compensation programs and the whole philosophy behind compensation in the caregiving business. As Noelle Driver, MD, says in the *AMA Journal of Ethics*, "Can clinicians of status care for patients in good faith without promoting good pay, benefits and organizational support for workers delivering care that is valued at a small fraction of their own?"[3]

When faced with an unpredictable volume of unfilled positions, the effect on compensation programs may lead to changes in the plan design. Companies forced to compete for scarce candidates may find that they must offer higher pay rates, referral or sign-on bonuses, retention bonuses and numerous other creative incentives to attract and hire the appropriate number and types of employees for the vacated positions. These are unforeseen changes that affect a compensation plan.

4.2 Compensation Design

There are various compensation program designs, including structured-based levels, step models, union compensation (based on a collective bargaining agreement), commission-based and others. The leadership team or consultant should determine the best type of design for the organization. Most medical practices do a hybrid model of market-based and traditional compensation-designed plans, sometimes with a step model included for various clinical positions.

Practice leadership must decide the compensation philosophy while designing the overall compensation structure. According to SHRM, a well-defined compensation philosophy supports the organization's strategic plan and initiatives, business goals, competitive outlook, operating objectives, as well as compensation and total reward strategies.[4] How the practice operates will direct the philosophy: If the practice desires equity, inclusiveness and transparent communication with the staff, the plan development process can reflect this by sharing the plan. While sharing the plan may seem overly transparent, one must consider the employees' perception of compensation planning.

Relevant Law

City ordinances, county regulations, along with state and federal laws can be a constraint when designing a compensation plan. All potentially relevant regulations should be considered. Some states, such as California, New York and others have implemented transparency laws requiring employers to post wage and salary information or at least make it available when requested.[5] As such, many of the online job boards post a salary range with the job posting. Creating a plan without considering legal requirements and regulations may result in legal disputes, fines or government intervention.

Some cities have significantly entrenched compensation benefits. For instance, San Francisco now requires all employers with 20 or more employees working eight or more hours a week to receive health coverage, part of the city's Health Care Security Ordinance.[6] Other cities may require paid sick leave or jury duty pay. These are items to be considered when designing any compensation plan. Legal counsel or a consultant familiar with applicable city ordinances can provide guidance on how to include them when planning.

Internet searches can offer information about city ordinances, county rules and state and federal laws. Search the county or city name and employment laws or regulations to become more familiar with these. State laws can be found by researching state and workforce commissions. Federal regulations can be found by visiting the websites for the Department of Labor, the Fair Labor Standards Act and the National Labor Relations Board. These websites and many others can provide considerable direction while developing the plan. Later in this book, Chapter 7 will discuss important relevant federal laws and provide valuable labor law resources.

Tax and Financial Considerations

Working with a certified accountant or business planner will prove helpful in developing the compensation plan. There are many factors to consider regarding tax implications and how the plan will affect a medical practice's financial viability. An employer may have tax requirements about which many healthcare executives may not be familiar. As benefits are reviewed, tax implications will be reviewed as well. Simply seeking professional tax counsel will provide ample information or direction.

If the organization operates under a collective bargaining agreement, the contract agreed upon between the employer and the employees' representation will address compensation, benefits and paid leave time. Complying with the collective bargaining agreement is required when designing compensation and benefits plans. Deviating from the contract without the union's consent may result in an unfair labor practice challenge or require further future negotiations. "The legal precedent for collective bargaining is one of the most important protected workers' rights in American law—and for good reason," notes Criterion, a global provider of human capital management software. "American employers are legally obligated to negotiate with unions in good faith."[7]

4.3 Compensation Planning

Compensation planning first involves the overall design, then the details, including what the organization will pay people, how it will develop various comp plans (such as aspects of salaried vs. non-salaried compensation) and more. A market analysis can be a helpful tool in determining effective compensation packages, especially in a dynamic and competitive market. To incorporate a market analysis into compensation planning, consider the following steps:[8]

- Define your compensation strategy
- Identify your benchmark jobs
- Collect and analyze market data
- Adjust your compensation packages

A compensation model is a structured framework that defines how an organization remunerates its employees, encompassing elements such as base salary, variable pay, benefits, equity and allowances. It serves to attract, retain and motivate talent while aligning with the organization's financial capacity and strategic goals. Compensation models can vary widely but are critical for balancing labor costs, complying with employment laws, and ensuring a competitive and equitable approach to rewarding employees, thereby contributing to talent management and organizational success. Below is an example of what a compensation model can look like for a physician.

Exhibit 4.1 MGMA Sample Compensation Model

Traditional cash net revenue compensation model		
Compensation elements	**Calculation**	**Compensation based on a primarily production-/volume-based arrangement**
Base compensation		
Physician—cash net revenue (CNR)		$600,000
Salary—annual draw		$200,000
Percent of net revenue received (minus annual salary draw)		45%
Total compensation to be paid based on CNR	$600,000 x .45 = $270,000	$270,000
Total compensation due minus annual salary draw	$270,000 - $200,000 = $70,000	$70,000
Quality compensation		
Quality metrics		$3,500
Value-based care payments (PMPM, shared savings, etc.)		$1,500
Total incentive/quality-based compensation	$3,500 + $1,500 = $5,000	$5,000
Total compensation	$270,000 + $5,000 = $275,000	**$275,000**

Taking these strategic steps can help your organization gain a comprehensive and balanced view of the market to align your pay rates while maintaining equity and consistency. When taking these steps, consider the different organizational levels when determining the right models.

Executive Compensation

The organization must consider many factors when developing an executive compensation plan. The plan needs to fit within the medical practice's overall operational structure. For the organization to attract and retain top talent, the plan must be designed to align with the business's goals.

The organization needs to determine what positions will be included in executive compensation plans. Tactically, executives make decisions, have a say in the organization's direction, design plans and strategies, and have responsibility for outcomes and goal attainment. "While executive compensation policies should never be a driving factor in forming healthcare operational strategy, it is important that strategy shapes and provides incentives to attract the right leaders to guide it," according to global auditing firm Grant Thornton.[9] The executive compensation program should be aligned with the executive's accountabilities, and compensation should be commensurate with attaining the goals of the business and its ultimate success.

Develop a communication strategy to recognize that executive compensation is not just the annualized salary of the staff member—it can include employment agreements, incentives, severance agreements, ownership possibilities and perquisites (perks). The organization should consider how top talent will respond to the executive compensation plan.

While designing the plan, consider what is appealing to top executives:

- Is the organization focused on outcomes and will executive compensation be tied to achieving them?
- If ownership or partnership is an option, can this be offered in place of some portion of direct payment?
- Could an executive receive extra compensation for exceeding expected results?
- Will executive compensation be tied to outcomes—win or lose?

- How will long-term results affect executive incentives and overall pay structure?

Most executives' ultimate concern is the overall compensation package, not just the annualized salary, which is advantageous for the organization and its executives as it will move both parties toward more outstanding accomplishments and remuneration. Address these items in the compensation structure to ensure a mutually beneficial "win."

Salaried Compensation

Salaried compensation means the employee is paid a set salary for work instead of being paid by the hour. Salaried employees receive a predetermined amount regardless of the number of hours worked in a pay period. Typically, salaried employees are exempt under the law, meaning they will not receive overtime pay.

Consider the employee's scope of work and responsibility to determine if they should receive a salary. The employee most likely will be salaried if the person:

- Is a manager or supervisor
- Conducts independent work
- Makes hiring or firing decisions
- Directs the business

The benefits to the organization of having salaried employees are that these employees generally work longer hours and are committed to the overall outcomes of the business, as opposed to simply finishing the work. Salaried employees typically enjoy the status of being salaried; it is a perception of both salaried and non-salaried employees that the salaried employee enjoys a higher standing than the hourly employee. "Salaried employees do not legally have to clock in and most employers don't require it," according to Bamboo HR, a human resources software company that helps businesses manage their employees. "This is because salaried employees are often offered a higher level of trust and accountability than hourly-paid employees."[10]

While it might seem advantageous to assign all salaried employees as exempt, some employees will not meet the requirements for exempt status.

Organizations can get into trouble categorizing employees as exempt who do not meet exempt or salaried guidelines. Consult the section in Chapter 7 on the U.S. Department of Labor's Fair Labor Standards Act (FLSA) for specific information on salaried employees.[11] Be sure to properly define the salaried employees and what job titles fall into this category and review these determinations annually. If the organization categorizes and pays people incorrectly, it will be subject to lawsuits and fines.

Non-Salaried Compensation

Non-salaried employees are hourly employees and are paid for the hours they work, not for the quality or outcome of the work. This designation also means the employee is eligible for overtime pay according to state or federal rules, whichever is stricter. All hours paid to hourly employees must be accounted for, documented and kept as a formal legal record, depending upon a state's rules.[12]

Job titles that fall under non-salaried compensation rules are typically:

- Support-type employees
- Back-office employees
- Clinical staff
- Hands-on staff
- Those who work task-oriented jobs

These employees generally are not on contract and do not have employment agreements.

Total Rewards and Compensation

The entirety of the business' overall compensation program is referred to as its total rewards package, which includes the salary, benefits, tuition reimbursement, relocation assistance and even loan forgiveness. The strategy of total rewards motivates employee commitment and loyalty and assists employees in understanding the organization and how their work contributes to attaining the goals and outcomes best for the business. "A total rewards program can be an effective tool in helping you meet these goals and distinguishing your business as an 'employer of choice,'" according to the Leavitt Group, an organization of affiliated independent insurance agencies.[13]

One strategy to help employees understand their total reward is to provide scenarios showing their complete compensation package. The scenarios should show the financial value of each item. Presenting employees a complete picture of their salary, benefits, perks, education assistance and advancement opportunities illustrates their job's value. Such a presentation is an effective strategy to recruit and retain employees.

These scenarios are also excellent tools during the negotiation phase of the recruitment process. If the business is competitive, demonstrating total compensation rewards will provide additional information for the candidate to make an informed decision. Most companies do not take the extra step of providing this information to potential employees. This tactic shows the candidate the straightforward approach the business takes with its employees. It also makes the case that the applicant will be highly valued should they choose the employment opportunity.

"One of the most important aspects of total rewards is how you communicate it internally," explains Paul Ashley of NFP, a benefits consultant. "Employers often do a great job making boardroom decisions about what benefits they're going to offer, but do a terrible job branding, marketing and communicating how an employee can take advantage of them."[14]

Present the total rewards to applicants and current employees in an easily understood manner. Often, candidates and employees need help understanding the total value of what a job offers. Ideally, review the scenario with the individual to explain the worth of each item. For example, explaining that the education reimbursement is worth $5,000 per year or that the business will assist the employee in obtaining a higher degree gives the candidate/employee a better understanding of the total compensation earned by staying or lost should they leave.

It is critical to be clear about where the organization's compensation plans rank in the market; remember that this strategy will only be effective if the business is competitive. The strategy will work to the organization's disadvantage if the pay or perks offered are below standard or compare unfavorably with competitors.

4.4 Benefits Plan Design and Program Administration

Identify the benefits plan and program clearly and design it to meet the objectives and goals of the organization. What is the purpose of the organization providing benefits to employees? The benefits strategy assists in the organization's overall competitiveness. Each organization should have an overall mission or vision for the benefits plan that supports the need to provide for employees' health and well-being. Approximately 80% of respondents to a survey conducted by the American Institute of CPAs said they would choose a job with benefits over an identical job with a 30% higher salary, but no benefits.[15]

Benefits affect the organization's overall budget, and there are also soft costs of benefits administration associated with recruitment and employee retention, and costs associated with such programs must be budgeted and reviewed periodically. In some businesses, the overall cost will not align with the strategy or end goals of the organization's bottom line, thus limiting the organization's offerings to the employees.

Partnering with a Benefits Broker

Depending on the organization's size, partnering with a benefits broker may be helpful. A healthcare or benefits broker assists the business in making better decisions, providing options and negotiating on the business's behalf to get the best benefits for their employees. The broker may also partner with outside entities to provide one-on-one counseling, enrollment, call center assistance and more extras for the employees. According to the Faison Group, a full-service insurance broker, benefits brokers should offer access to a wide range of carriers and be open to assisting with claims, as well as maintaining compliance with HIPAA and other legislation.[16] Additionally, brokers can dissect the plan utilization and provide in-depth reports and an overview of the programs, which is especially worthwhile if the organization needs to increase or decrease coverage. If programs are underutilized, a broker can help design a communication strategy and offer alternatives for the future.

The broker should offer services such as workforce analysis, determining the needs of the workforce based on age, gender, nationality and various identifiers that establish possible desires of employees. When designing the benefits plan, determine what the employees need and want. Also, consider what direct and indirect competitors offer. Look at surrounding businesses that may pull existing employees. What do they offer, and what is more appealing about their workplace benefits? Employee response and direction will directly result in employees having more buy-in and commitment.

Review the benefits plan annually or more often to meet employer requirements and employees' wants. During the review process, consider the affordability of the benefits offered:

- Are costs increasing?
- How much of the expense should employees bear?
- How much should the organization absorb?

This review allows the employer to consider the needs of the business balanced with the employees' needs and desires.

The government has been known to dictate changes or requirements to an employer's health plan or other benefits. The Affordable Care Act required employers with 50 or more employees to provide insurance to employees or pay penalties.[17] Some businesses determined it was worthwhile financially not to offer insurance but to advise employees to seek the public insurance option. Companies that used this option paid fines based on several factors set forth by the government.

Communicating the plan to employees is part of the overall strategy and essential to understanding employees' needs. The government has various requirements for communicating benefits plans to employees, but the basic disclosure statements need to be revised for effective recruitment and retention. Effectively communicating thorough knowledge of benefits offered provides an excellent opportunity to improve employee engagement. "Getting employee feedback, whether it be through surveys or one-on-one talks with staff, will help you narrow down the list of benefits that your company should be targeting," according to Embroker, a digitally-native business insurance company.[18] Explaining to employees how the organization cares for them, is eager to keep them healthy, and encourages them to participate in the benefits creates strong relationships between the organization and the employees.

The administration of the benefits plan involves managing the employee benefits programs. The administration may fall under human resources, payroll or accounting, depending on the organization's size. Some organizations outsource the benefits administration. When determining which department the administration falls under, consider how it is best handled and how the employees perceive it. For instance, placing administration under payroll may communicate to the employees that it is a logistical function, not an employee relations function.

Administering the benefits program involves maintaining who is eligible for benefits, collecting monthly or biweekly contributions and paying for benefits. It also involves:

- Enrollments
- Terminations
- Reconciliations
- Correspondence
- Education
- Training

The role of the benefits administration team is essential to communicate about the benefits and maintain compliance and efficiency of the program administration.

There are many software programs and platforms available to administer benefits. Many payrolls, human resources and accounting systems include benefits administration as a function of the software or platform. Established providers such as ADP, Paychex and Justworks offer integrated solutions which can manage voluntary benefits through payroll deductions, personalize employee benefit decisions and make it easier for employees to self-manage open enrollment periods or make other personal changes to coverage.[19] No matter how small the benefit offerings are, all benefits administration should be part of the technology structure.

4.5 Competitiveness

As reviewed earlier, the benefits strategy assists the organization's overall competitiveness. Some benefits that provide additional competitiveness are matching retirement, automotive assistance or a nurse care hotline. Some benefit options are entirely voluntary to the employee, and voluntary plans can be offered as a bundle or provided separately. Some examples are:

- Disability insurance
- Life insurance
- Critical illness
- Pet insurance
- Legal helpline
- Accident insurance
- Dental or vision insurance

Nearly half of employees responding to a Voya Financial survey indicated they were also more likely to stay with their employer if offered access to voluntary benefits including disability income coverage, critical illness insurance or accident insurance.[20] According to Voya, in 2022 there was a 41% increase in employers offering voluntary benefits and a 16% increase in employees eligible for them.

While the appeal of voluntary insurance for the employer is obvious—less outlay and the appearance of offerings—it may also be seen as not providing for the employee or, worse yet, being cheap. It is essential to determine how these decisions will be perceived.

Systems and Processes for Benefits and Compensation

Employers should develop a system and process to set up, maintain and administer benefits, compensation, time off and paid and unpaid leave. Appropriate processes, such as monthly or quarterly reporting, maintain the programs' validity and offer legitimacy. The onus is on the employer to provide a structure to track, notify and report information to the government, leadership, employees and managers.

The federal and some state governments set forth regulations for health insurance or benefits offerings. Whichever department administers the benefits must be familiar with all rules and regulations, legal requirements and specifications for the benefits offered. Compliance with benefits plans is a requirement and a non-negotiable for the business.

Employers who offer health insurance and have more than 20 employees must provide COBRA coverage to employees.[21] COBRA, the Consolidated Omnibus Budget Reconciliation Act, allows employees, former employees and their families protection from losing their health coverage. This protection will enable employees to retain the insurance and pay the premiums post-termination.

Moreover, the business must be familiar with HIPAA, The Health Insurance Portability and Accountability Act of 1996, "a federal law that required the creation of national standards to protect sensitive patient health information from being disclosed without the patient's consent or knowledge."[22]

4.6 Health and Wellness

Making a priority of employees' overall health and wellness will give the organization a competitive edge and create better engagement with employees. Employee wellness has become a hot topic in recent years as it directly relates to employee job satisfaction. "Increasing the various types of wellness boosts employee performance and productivity in a big way," according to Workhuman, a cloud-based company that provides human capital management software solutions. "And wellness programs aren't beneficial for employees only. They also benefit managers, teams and organizations as a whole."[23]

Wellness offerings may include:

- Education on preventable health conditions
- Wellness activities such as weight loss programs, smoking cessation programs and risk assessments
- Training or education in first aid and CPR
- Wellness checks
- Onsite health screenings or offsite screenings that may relate to increased healthcare utilization and decreased chronic diseases

Additional wellness benefits include employee assistance programs, therapy or counseling, sick care onsite, stress reduction programs, quiet rooms, therapy, massage programs and onsite exercise programs. Discounts for off-site programs and incentives related to gifts or cash rewards are also popular. Overall, these benefits may assist the employer by decreasing the need for health insurance.

Employees enduring financial challenges may also see increased stress levels that could correlate to less productivity at work. According to the Financial Industry Regulatory Authority, about two thirds of the American population is also considered financially illiterate.[24] Offering money management classes, financial solvency classes or financial assistance or advice through outside fiscal management resources will benefit employees. Educational opportunities focused on money or cost savings are also a perk for employees directly related to their wellness.

Paid and Unpaid Time Off

Many employees may believe that employers are required to offer paid time off for all holidays, illnesses and leaves of absence. However, unless required by a state or local law as outlined below, like other benefits an employer may choose to offer, paid time off is a matter of budget and competitiveness as a desirable employer.[25]

Exhibit 4.2 PTO Accrual Rate

Years of Service	Total PTO Days
0-2	17
3-5	19
6-10	24
11-15	29
16+	34

Holidays

Businesses are not required to provide paid federal or bank holidays.[26] Federal or bank holidays include:

- New Year's Day
- Martin Luther King Jr Day
- Presidents Day
- Memorial Day
- Independence Day
- Labor Day
- Columbus Day
- Thanksgiving
- Christmas Day

There may be other state or city holidays, and employers should check with the state or city/county for requirements.

Exhibit 4.3 PTO Accrual Rates Per Years of Service

Years of Service	Total PTO Days	Paid Holidays	Total
0-2	15	7	22
3-5	20	7	27
6-10	25	7	32
11-15	30	7	37
16+	35	7	42

Sick Time

There is no federal requirement to offer sick time or sick leave.[27] There may be a state, county or city regulation or law governing sick time. Sick time is for an employee to recover from an illness or injury or care for ill relatives. In the case of caring for a loved one, there are various eligibility requirements and potential claims for discrimination that may arise.

When developing the policy, guidelines or a handbook regarding sick time, it is best to consider employee and business needs when releasing the policy. In some organizations, attendance policies encourage employees to work sick, but this is a dangerous policy that may eventually work against the organization. "This gap in worker protections has severe consequences: it increases the spread of infectious disease, prevents workers and their families from accessing healthcare and harms businesses and the overall economy," notes A Better Balance, a national nonprofit legal advocacy organization dedicated to work-family justice.[28] Review the punitive nature of a policy and determine the best way to encourage employees to care for themselves if sick.

Time Off

According to Indeed, a paid time-off policy affects more than just the employer and the employee: "While employees appreciate the paid time off to spend on vacations and personal time, they also need this time to maintain a healthy work-life balance. Allowing your employees to take paid time off may actually benefit their mental and physical health. Employees who work long hours may have increased absenteeism due to unexpected illnesses and injuries, which can cause employers to actually lose money in the long run."[29]

A written time-off policy should include what will be paid and will not be paid, how many days are allowed, the process to request and the consequences of excessive time off. The time-off policy should be part of the employee handbook and new employee orientation. Also the time-off request form should overview the time-off policy on paper or online. If the company offers paid time off, employees should be informed via their paystub how many hours or days are available to them, how many they have used and how many remain. Some employers choose to have sick time, holiday and vacation in a lump sum called "Paid Time Off." In this case, it must be identified and explained in writing.

Regulated Leaves

Various leaves governed by federal or state, or county governments are available to employees. Here are two of them.

1. The Family and Medical Leave Act (FMLA) allows employees who meet eligibility requirements to have unpaid leave that affords the employee job protection.[30] Employees must meet various eligibility conditions, such as being employed for one year and having worked 1,250 hours (about one month and three weeks). Employees must also receive a

physician's certification for medical leave. FMLA only affects employers having 50 or more employees.

2. All employers must provide leave to employees having military obligations under U.S.ERRA (Uniformed Services Employment and Reemployment Rights Act).[31]

There may be other state or city holidays, and employers should check with the state or city/county for requirements. In general, the key to any payment or benefits is that whatever is done for one employee must be done for all in the same class or group of employees.

4.7 Practice in Action

Marie Eslick, Human Resources Director at Ohio's Apex Dermatology and Skin Center, worked with her carrier and broker to carve out lower rates, with additional assistance from Apex management. "Once we did that, the spouse coverage and the family coverage went through the roof, because people saw the difference in price. It was still good coverage and it'd be more affordable, so we definitely got more people on board."

Eslick also worked to add an all-new voluntary benefits package, partnering with ADP as a benefits management platform. "We even added lifestyle benefits … there's various different discount platforms out there that you can put in place for your folks that are no cost to you. So I added two of those," she says. The ADP platform, she adds, gave the employees more centralized information and control over their benefits, as well as a better variety of voluntary benefits and discounts. "I always tell folks here, if you are going on a vacation, buying a car, or even going to the movies or a sporting event, there's a discount out there, you should be using it. So all those lifestyle discounts add to the program as well."

Eslick says those enhanced benefits have been critical in both attracting and retaining staff in a competitive healthcare market. "In the Greater Cleveland area, you have two huge hospital systems that you're competing with, and although we'll never match their medical, dental and vision, we knew that we could get pretty close to it. And we offer some additional things that they don't have for their employees. So that definitely makes a difference when we start to talk to people, even just in the interview stage, about the discounts and benefits that we have. We even give discounts for aesthetic services for our associates, plus a friends and family discount."

Ultimately, the mix of both traditional and non-traditional benefits helps differentiate Apex and provide an added draw for employees. "People really see the difference and get excited about being part of a company that has such a wealth of different benefit options. And that has definitely helped not only retaining people, but also in our recruitment efforts."

Eslick says something as simple as Apex's working hours can also be a draw for employees. "One of the things we can offer that a hospital does not is a schedule that is pretty much Monday to Friday, 8-5. Hospitals now are really looking for evenings and weekends, and they're 24/7. So we're able to pull some of those folks because of the benefit of having a family-life balance. So we kind of include that as a benefit, as well."

4.8 Summary

The overall success of your organization depends on the happiness and well-being of your workers, and appropriate compensation and benefits are a major piece of that puzzle. As other industries become more competitive in terms of pay and other benefits packages, healthcare HR managers need to recognize the value of a flexible and well-designed benefits plan.

Key points discussed in this chapter include:

- Compensation planning at all levels must be designed in a competitive fashion. How an organization operates will help guide the comprehensive compensation plan and structure.
- A robust benefits strategy assists in an organization's overall competitiveness. It should be designed with an organization's objectives and goals in mind. Working with a benefits broker can help a practice develop their benefits strategy by providing options and negotiating on the business's behalf to get the best benefits for their employees.

- Prioritizing employees' overall health and wellness will give the organization a competitive edge in the job market and create better engagement with current employees.
- Communicating the benefits plan to employees is part of the overall strategy and essential to understanding employees' needs. This also provides an excellent opportunity to improve employee engagement with potential for feedback on types of benefits the organization should target.
- The key to any payment or benefits program is that whatever is done for one employee must be done for all in the same class or group of employees. When developing the policy, guidelines or a handbook regarding sick time, it is best to consider employee and business needs when releasing the policy.

In the next chapter, we will discuss the importance of the pre-employment and onboarding process in setting expectations and welcoming employees for an extended stay.

Notes

1. Brookings. https://www.brookings.edu/articles/essential-but-undervalued-millions-of-health-care-workers-arent-getting-the-pay-or-respect-they-deserve-in-the-covid-19-pandemic/

2. Wolters Kluwer. https://www.wolterskluwer.com/en/expert-insights/working-at-a-hospital-vs-private-practice-whats-right-for-you

3. *AMA Journal of Ethics.* https://journalofethics.ama-assn.org/article/what-do-we-owe-health-care-workers-who-earn-low-wages/2022-09

4. SHRM. https://www.shrm.org/resourcesandtools/tools-and-samples/toolkits/pages/buildingamarket-basedpaystructurefromscratch.aspx

5. Gibson Dunn. https://www.gibsondunn.com/new-york-state-enacts-pay-transparency-law/

6. City and County of San Francisco. https://sf.gov/information/understanding-health-care-security-ordinance

7. Criterion. https://www.criterionhcm.com/white-papers/cba-payroll-changes

8. LinkedIn. https://www.linkedin.com/advice/0/how-do-you-determine-effective-compensation-packages-o50mf

9. Grant Thornton. https://www.grantthornton.com/insights/articles/health-care/2023/securing-balance-in-healthcare-executive-compensation

10. Bamboo HR. https://www.bamboohr.com/resources/hr-glossary/salaried-employee

11. U.S. Department of Labor. https://webapps.dol.gov/elaws/whd/flsa/screen75.asp

12. Paychex. https://www.paychex.com/articles/payroll-taxes/whats-the-difference-between-exempt-and-non-exempt-employees

13. Leavitt Group. https://news.leavitt.com/human-resources-benefits/total-rewards-program/

14. Marathon Health. https://www.marathon-health.com/blog/how-total-rewards-strategies-are-changing-hr-today/

15. AICPA. https://www.aicpa-cima.com/news/article/americans-favor-workplace-benefits-4-to-1-over-extra-salary-aicpa-survey

16. Faison Group. https://www.faisongroup.com/about-us/blog/2015/07/10-things-your-benefits-broker-should-be-doing/

17. U.S. Department of Health and Human Services. https://www.hhs.gov/healthcare/about-the-aca/index.html

18. Embroker. https://www.embroker.com/blog/how-to-design-an-employee-benefits-program/

19. ADP. https://www.adp.com/what-we-offer/benefits/benefits-administration.aspx

20. Voya Financial. https://www.voya.com/voya-insights/voluntary-benefits-101-what-are-they-and-how-do-they-work

21. DOL. https://www.dol.gov/general/topic/health-plans/cobra

22. CDC. https://www.cdc.gov/phlp/publications/topic/hipaa.html

23. Workhuman. https://www.workhuman.com/blog/benefits-of-wellness-programs/

24. Corporate Finance Institute. https://corporatefinanceinstitute.com/resources/management/financial-literacy/

25. DOL. https://www.dol.gov/general/topic/workhours/vacation_leave

26. U.S. Department of Commerce. https://www.commerce.gov/hr/practitioners/compensation-policies/premium-pay/eligibility-for-paid-holidays

27. DOL. https://www.dol.gov/general/topic/workhours/sickleave

28. A Better Balance. https://www.abetterbalance.org/sick-without-a-safety-net/

29. Indeed. https://www.indeed.com/hire/c/info/how-to-create-a-paid-time-off-policy

30. DOL. https://www.dol.gov/agencies/whd/fmla

31. DOL. https://www.dol.gov/agencies/vets/programs/userra/U.S.ERRA-Pocket-Guide

Chapter 5

Pre-Employment,
Interviewing and Onboarding

5.1 Hiring Processes and Systems
in the Pre-Employment Phase

The post-pandemic Great Resignation spawned a movement among workers known as "quiet quitting," which saw many employees come to work but neglect their assigned duties mostly due to feeling not engaged.[1] But a more lasting trend called "quick quitting" ought to have HR professionals more concerned. According to the 2022 *Job Seeker Nation* report, 1-in-3 new hires is likely to quit their job within 90 days if their responsibilities, management or benefits fail to live up to the promises made as they were hired.[2]

This chapter will discuss various strategies and techniques that can help keep employees engaged and committed to their new positions, from the moment they see an online job listing to their first day on the job and beyond. Employee turnover is inevitable. But it can have a silver lining if the medical practice approaches the hiring process as not just filling a position that has become vacant but instead as an opportunity to examine the organization and effect improvements wherever possible. As seen with the "quick quitting" phenomenon, role clarity and picking the right candidate are essential when filling vacancies, especially in the stressful world of a healthcare workplace.

HR departments should strive to follow a consistent system for the hiring processes of pre-employment, interviewing and onboarding to ensure all essential tasks are addressed with each new hire to make all go smoothly. Consistency of practice is vital to ensure that required elements of the hiring process are executed appropriately to avoid inadvertently violating labor law. Laws surrounding employment are numerous and often complicated, as will be discussed in Chapter 7. Continuing culture requires constant definition and addition of new laws; therefore, HR should carefully check federal and state laws and remain up to date with all labor and employment laws. It is further mandatory that laws applicable to the practice are understood and that the application of the laws is equitable and carefully applied. The essential idea is that the practice should know how laws are applied to protect the practice and its employees.

Depending on the size of the medical practice, it may be wise to invest in a human resource technology system, commonly referred to as a human resources management system (HRMS). According to SHRM, these management systems are used to store employee information and support various HR functions, such as benefits, payroll and training.[3] HRMSs assist with workforce management to recruit, hire, manage, develop and engage employees, onboard employees and manage both performance and compensation.

5.2 Pre-Employment

For this discussion, pre-employment includes all activities prior to acceptance of an employment offer by a selected candidate.

Exhibit 5.1 Pre-employment Process

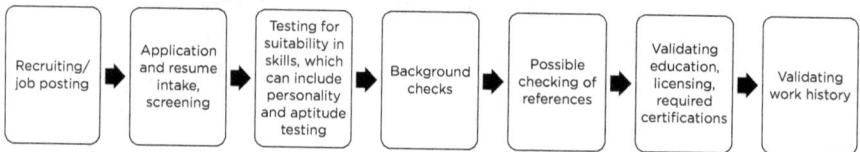

Recruiting/job posting → Application and resume intake, screening → Testing for suitability in skills, which can include personality and aptitude testing → Background checks → Possible checking of references → Validating education, licensing, required certifications → Validating work history

Avoiding Discrimination in Pre-Employment Activities

One of the most effective ways to ensure sound employee selection procedures and to avoid unlawful discrimination is for medical practices to carefully develop job-related position descriptions outlining job duties along with required skills and abilities for each position, then posting only those elements on internal or external job postings.

Employers may elicit adequate information on their employment applications to aid in making a good selection. They should ask only about specific job requirements and relevant skills required to perform a particular job. "To protect yourself, you need to make sure that you clearly understand what information you're legally allowed to request from candidates, and how much of it they are required by law to disclose," explains GMS, a benefits administrator.[4]

It is essential that employers carefully examine the job-relatedness of all questions and develop different employment applications for different job groups, if appropriate. In screening employment applicants, assumptions should not be made based on an applicant's identity or status. For example, an employer should not assume that because a woman has small children, that the candidate cannot work odd hours. The applicant should be asked if working odd hours is acceptable, without regard to parenting status.

Employers are advised to check applicable federal laws, discussed in Chapter 7, such as Title VII of the Civil Rights Act of 1964, and local and state laws for the practice location.[5]

A sound selection process aims to obtain good employees who meet specific work requirements and perform particular job duties. Although an organization should aim to have a diverse candidate pool, a person's race, sex, sexual orientation, disability, color, religion, age, genetic information, national origin or gender identity are not indicators of an individual's potential to be a good worker and should not be part of the interview discussion.

HR professionals are usually familiar with federal anti-discrimination statutes—such as Title VII of the Civil Rights Act of 1964—but they also must be aware of similar state laws that may provide more protections for workers. Employers are advised to inform hiring managers on what they can and cannot ask interviewees or the appropriate way to phrase certain questions during interviews, according to the federal laws and the laws of the employer's respective state.

Selection Criteria

Several steps should guide the selection criteria before the interviewing process begins:

1. Validating the need for a position and its qualifications
2. Creating the job posting
3. Intake of applications
4. Review of the applications
5. After reviewing the applications and careful consideration, narrow the applications down to the few that seem the most appropriate and reach out to the most promising potential interviewee
6. Once all steps are completed, informed interviewing should begin.

Hiring Using AI

Artificial Intelligence (AI) is increasingly being utilized in the hiring process within medical practices. AI-powered applicant tracking systems (ATS) can screen resumes, identify qualified candidates and match them to job requirements, saving HR professionals valuable time and effort. However, there are some concerns when relying only on AI to get candidates to the hiring managers. Some drawbacks include:

- Lack of human judgment needed to assess intangible qualities such as cultural fit, soft skills and emotional intelligence, which are crucial in healthcare settings.
- AI may struggle to understand the unique context and requirements of medical practices, leading to mismatches

between candidate qualifications and organizational needs.

- Overreliance on AI-driven automation in hiring may lead to "automation bias," where HR professionals defer too much to algorithmic decisions without critical evaluation or consideration of alternative perspectives.
- AI may overlook relevant factors such as career transitions, personal experiences, or gaps in employment history, which could be important in assessing a candidate's suitability for a medical practice role.
- If AI algorithms make errors or produce biased outcomes, it can be challenging to identify and correct these issues, potentially leading to unfair treatment of candidates and damage to the organization's reputation.

While AI can be a valuable tool in the hiring process, it's essential for medical practices to implement safeguards, ensure transparency, and complement AI with human judgment to mitigate potential risks and maximize its effectiveness in selecting the best candidates.

5.3 Interviewing

Effective interviewing uncovers essential data from the potential employee, which is valuable when the hiring decision-making begins. A well-conducted interview is the healthcare employer's side of a two-sided conversation guided by specific, carefully planned strategies. "The personal interview is your chance to really get to know your prospective employees—you'll be delving deeper into the skills and requirements you've noted on the resume and phone screening," according to the *Hartford Business Owner's Playbook*.[6] "Mostly, the interview allows you to get a sense of the intangibles, such as passion, initiative, goals, cultural fit, attitudes and communication skills." In a broad sense, the interview is necessary for those engaged to exchange information to evaluate compatibility. Several key practices should come into play:

Preparation: Thorough preparation in anticipation of the interview is necessary for the interview to go smoothly and garner the information needed between parties.

Presentation: Employers should strive to be creative in presenting the job opportunity and the interview questions while designing and presenting information to foster an understanding of the position along with its requirements to help gauge the applicant's competence and cultural fit. Listen carefully to the interviewee's responses and other comments. Remember that the candidate is also interviewing the practice.

Learn about the interviewee's career goals: According to Indeed, asking general questions about a candidate's professional interests along with why they're interested in the position can give you an opportunity to understand their expectations of professional development, and assess their understanding of the practice and the position itself.[7]

Build comfortable communication: Essential to the rapport-building exercise is that distractions such as phones or others should be removed from the interview location.

Open opportunity for applicants' questions: Encourage applicants to ask questions and give them time to ask them. Applicants' questions can be very telling.

Manage direction and flow of the interview: It is likewise important for the interviewer to refrain from allowing lapses in conversation or too many moments of silence. As well, be careful not to conduct an interview that seems rushed. Carefully managing the direction of the interview and the smooth flow it should take helps the interviewer and the potential employee. Always remember that communication is equally vital to the interviewee and the interviewer.

Active listening: A skillful interviewer carefully guides the conversation with active listening—asking pertinent questions in a supportive tone and possibly offering a brief summary of certain pieces of information that the applicant gives. "Listen more, talk less … the interview is mostly about the applicant, so listen attentively," according to the *Hartford Playbook*. "Also, note if they have done their homework about your company."

SAMPLE INTERVIEW QUESTIONS FOR CLINICAL POSITIONS

When interviewing candidates for clinical positions in a medical practice, such as nurses, medical assistants, or laboratory technicians, it's essential to assess their clinical expertise, patient care skills, communication abilities, and adherence to healthcare regulations. Ask follow-up questions to delve deeper into the candidate's clinical expertise, experience, and problem-solving abilities. Consider conducting practical assessments or scenario-based questions to gauge their clinical skills in real-life situations.

Here are some interview questions to help you evaluate candidates:

1. Can you describe your experience and qualifications in clinical healthcare roles, including any relevant certifications or licenses?
   - This question allows candidates to provide an overview of their clinical background and credentials.

2. What motivated you to pursue a career in clinical healthcare, and why are you interested in working in a medical practice specifically?
   - This question assesses the candidate's motivation and alignment with the practice's goals.

3. How do you ensure patient safety and infection control in a clinical setting?
   - This question evaluates the candidate's understanding of safety protocols and adherence to healthcare regulations.

4. Can you describe your experience with electronic health records (EHR) or healthcare information systems?
   - This question assesses the candidate's familiarity with technology used in healthcare settings.

5. How do you approach patient assessments and care planning in a clinical setting?
   - This question evaluates the candidate's clinical judgment and care planning abilities.

6. Can you provide an example of a challenging patient care situation you've encountered and how you handled it?
   - This question assesses the candidate's problem-solving skills and ability to manage complex patient scenarios.

7. Communication is vital in healthcare. How do you ensure effective communication with patients, their families, and other members of the healthcare team?
   - This question evaluates the candidate's interpersonal and communication skills.

8. How do you prioritize tasks and manage your workload in a fast-paced clinical environment?
   - This question assesses the candidate's ability to handle the demands of a busy medical practice.

9. In a clinical role, you may encounter patients with diverse backgrounds and needs. How do you approach cultural competence and sensitivity in patient care?
   - This question assesses the candidate's awareness of cultural competence and their commitment to providing culturally sensitive care.

10. How do you stay updated with the latest healthcare guidelines, best practices, and industry trends relevant to your clinical role?
    - This question evaluates the candidate's commitment to ongoing learning and professional development.

11. Can you describe your experience with medical equipment and instruments relevant to your clinical role?
    - This question assesses the candidate's technical skills and familiarity with clinical tools.

12. How do you handle emergencies or unexpected medical situations, and what steps do you take to ensure patient safety during such incidents?
    - This question evaluates the candidate's ability to remain composed and respond effectively in critical situations.

13. Can you provide an example of a time when you collaborated successfully with other healthcare professionals, such as physicians or nurses, to deliver patient care?
    - This question assesses the candidate's teamwork and collaboration skills.

14. Are you comfortable with administering medications or treatments, if relevant to the role? Can you describe your experience in medication administration?
    - This question evaluates the candidate's knowledge of medication safety and administration procedures.

15. What do you find most rewarding about working in a clinical role in a medical practice, and how do you contribute to ensuring a positive patient experience?
    - This question allows candidates to express their commitment to patient care and satisfaction.

Inspiring healthcare excellence.

MGMA

SAMPLE INTERVIEW QUESTIONS FOR
FRONT OFFICE STAFF IN A MEDICAL PRACTICE

When interviewing candidates for a front office staff position in a medical practice, it's important to assess their interpersonal skills, attention to detail, organizational abilities, and their ability to handle patient interactions professionally. Remember to probe further with follow-up questions to gain a deeper understanding of the candidate's qualifications and suitability for the role. Additionally, consider including scenario-based questions to assess problem-solving skills in practical situations.

Here are some interview questions to help you evaluate candidates:

1. **Can you describe your previous experience in a medical front office role?**
   - This question allows candidates to provide an overview of their relevant experience and qualifications.

2. **How do you handle a busy front desk with multiple patients checking in and out simultaneously?**
   - This question assesses the candidate's ability to multitask and stay organized during peak times.

3. **Patient confidentiality is crucial in healthcare. How do you ensure the privacy and security of patient information?**
   - This question evaluates the candidate's understanding of HIPAA regulations and their commitment to patient privacy.

4. **Can you describe a time when you had to deal with an upset or difficult patient? How did you handle the situation?**
   - This question assesses the candidate's interpersonal skills and their ability to handle challenging patient interactions.

5. **What software or electronic health record (EHR) systems are you familiar with, and how proficient are you in using them?**
   - This question evaluates the candidate's technical skills and familiarity with healthcare software.

6. **How do you prioritize tasks when faced with multiple responsibilities at the front desk?**
   - This question assesses the candidate's ability to manage their workload effectively and prioritize tasks.

7. **Can you provide an example of a situation where you had to work as part of a team in a healthcare setting?**
   - This question evaluates the candidate's teamwork and collaboration skills.

8. **Accuracy is essential in maintaining patient records. How do you ensure that you enter data correctly and minimize errors?**
   - This question assesses the candidate's attention to detail and commitment to maintaining accurate records.

9. **How would you handle a situation where a patient arrived late for their appointment and was upset about the wait time?**
   - This question assesses the candidate's problem-solving and customer service skills.

10. **In a medical practice, you may have to handle insurance-related inquiries from patients. How comfortable are you with insurance verification and explaining insurance coverage to patients?**
    - This question evaluates the candidate's knowledge of insurance processes and their ability to communicate effectively with patients regarding insurance matters.

11. **Can you describe any experience you have with scheduling appointments, managing calendars, or coordinating patient appointments with multiple providers?**
    - This question assesses the candidate's scheduling and organizational skills.

12. **Why do you want to work in a medical practice, and what do you find most rewarding about this type of role?**
    - This question allows candidates to express their motivation and passion for working in a healthcare setting.

13. **How do you stay updated with changes in medical office procedures, regulations, or industry trends?**
    - This question evaluates the candidate's commitment to professional development and staying informed about the healthcare industry.

14. **Are you comfortable handling billing inquiries or financial transactions at the front desk, and do you have any experience in this area?**
    - This question assesses the candidate's financial and billing knowledge, if applicable to the role.

15. **Can you provide an example of a time when you went above and beyond to provide exceptional service to a patient or customer?**
    - This question helps assess the candidate's commitment to delivering outstanding patient care and customer service.

Inspiring
healthcare
excellence.™

MGMA

5.4 Making the Offer

Before making an offer, avoid costly mistakes with a thorough reference check and background check, or at least make the offer contingent on the reference and background check. According to a Resume Lab survey, 56% of applicants surveyed admitted they had misrepresented themselves on their resume, including work experience, education, skills or job duties.[8] Conducting a legal, consistent and fair background check process that is the same for every candidate can help prevent issues before an offer is made, according to GoodHire, a background check company. "A background check can verify someone's work history, experience and education; uncover lies or omissions; and reveal a criminal history."[9] A background check policy needs to indicate:

- What types of background checks will be conducted and for whom
- How background check results will affect employment decisions
- When background checks will be conducted

Once the decision concerning the successful candidate has been made, prepare for the discussion: script it with key messages; prepare for the salary discussion in case they want to negotiate; and ensure that the practice can persuade the candidate on why they should accept its offer.

5.5 Onboarding

Since the early 19th century, onboarding has become a necessity in the workplace to efficiently and effectively integrate new employees into the workplace.[10] Onboarding brings new employees into the organization by providing information, training, mentoring and coaching during their first 6-12 months of employment. It helps new employees more quickly contribute to the organization, increase their comfort level, reinforce their decision to join the organization and enhance productivity. It also encourages employee commitment, engagement and retention.

But it has to be done correctly and thoughtfully. According to a Gallup study, one in five employees report that their most recent onboarding was poor, or they received no onboarding at all.[11] Onboarding should fulfill the promises made during the hiring process and lay the foundation for long-term engagement and performance. Gallup further suggests onboarding should answer five questions employees will have about the employer and its culture:

Exhibit 5.3 Five Questions Onboarding Should Answer

"What do we believe in around here?"	"What are my strengths?"	"What is my role?"	"Who are my partners?"	"What does my future look like?"
• The way you explain your benefits, time off and other policies and what those policies actually are, will help new employees far more than handouts explaining "core value". • Employers should consider how their culture is experienced and expressed during the onboarding process.	• Employees need to know what they do best, and where their skills can be best put to use. Learning and developing those strengths suggests an employer wants to know about their workers and see them succeed in the long term.	• There's often a significant difference between external and internal job postings and descriptions, and the work that actually needs to be done – with only 50% of employees strongly suggesting they know what is expected of them at work. • Managers play the most important role in setting expectations for new employees.	• As the phenomenon of home-based employment continues to wane, new employees seek socialization. And while they may feel warmly welcomed in the first week, they may feel isolated and lost three months into the job. • Managers can build the important connections and help with relationship-building opportunities, proactively expanding a new employee's social network by making introductions and through other advocacy efforts	• Onboarding offers managers the opportunity to help employees see opportunities to learn and grow. Professional development can be built into the job experience when a pathway is outlined.

Research has also demonstrated that onboarding reduces stress and the chance of employees quitting soon after starting more than a traditional orientation program. "A well-designed, fun and engaging onboarding process has a significantly greater effect on employee engagement and retention compared to the old-school mentality of one-day orientation," says Ben Peterson of Bamboo HR.[12] Onboarding and new employee orientation programs help employees develop their identity within the organization and adopt a team spirit, which contribute to healthy attitudes toward the practice and can lower absenteeism and employee turnover.

Onboarding and new employee orientation programs are highly effective ways to communicate that the practice demands full effort from its staff to maximize productivity and the quality of services and that the practice values and respects its employees. They also inform new hires about the practice's policy prohibiting unlawful discrimination and harassment. Keep in mind that a practice's website gives the first impression of the organization, followed by the interview process and then the type of new employee orientation program the practice offers. All these influences affect newly hired employees' long-term commitment to the practice. According to the *HBR*, companies which implement a formal onboarding program can see a 50% greater employee retention rate and 62% more productivity from those new employees.[13]

Benefits of a well-organized programs include:[14]

- Reduces time it takes for employee to become productive and minimizes errors
- Ensures employee is aware and is in compliance with organization's policies, procedures and expectations
- Improved job satisfaction as employees feel supported and engaged from the beginning. It is suggested to have regular check-ins throughout the new employee's first year.

Before Onboarding

A potentially awkward time gap for new employees occurs after accepting a new job offer and the start date for the new job. That window can be as short as a few days, typically between 2-4 weeks, but in the case of physicians or other providers, as long as a few months. This lag time may create employee remorse in taking a job with a new employer, and most employers overlook this time as an opportunity to build early engagement with the new hire.

Potential strategies to help with the gap between hiring and start date while diminishing the chances of remorse setting in might include the following:

- Text message, phone call or other form of communication from the office manager confirming that the practice has the correct information for the new hire

- Formal email 5-7 days before the new employee's start date confirming such details as arrival time on the first day, the address of the location if there are multiple sites, any documentation the employee might need to bring to set up employment with the new group or anything else necessary for the first day

In a competitive job environment, a little outreach can go a long way. A call from the supervisor could set the stage for how a new employee will be treated at the new job. Some practices send welcoming packages to the new employee's home as a welcome gift. This could be as simple as a branded merchandise with the practice name on it. Either way, outreach lets the employee know your practice is excited to have them.

Initial Onboarding

Notably, a medical practice's orientation program should consist of two distinct parts: a general organizational overview and a departmental orientation. Ideally, orientation should be scheduled during the new hire's first work week. The organizational overview should provide information on the practice's history, mission, values, policies, compensation and benefits. In addition, the general overview should introduce the practice's strategic plan and structure. This part should be given by the HR department or a person responsible for these activities.

The orientation program's frequency depends on the practice's size, employee turnover and the number of new employees. In a small practice, employee orientation may be conducted individually as new employees are hired, and the person responsible for employee administration usually conducts the orientation. Medium-sized practices might offer this program once every few months, whereas larger practices may hold these programs more often.

The benefits of orientation, according to AIRH, can be fundamentally important: reducing the stress and anxiety of new hires, increasing productivity and decreasing mistakes, reducing turnover and contributing to a positive relationship and better communication between the new employee, their manager and their coworkers.[15]

5.6 Reviewing the Employee Handbook and Orientation

An employee handbook is distributed to all the group's employees and includes summary descriptions referencing management's HR policies and procedures. An employee handbook provides an overview and a vehicle for explaining and familiarizing employees with the medical practice's history, values, expectations, acceptable behavior, benefit programs, employee responsibilities and so on. All employees should have access to a physical copy of the employee handbook or be directed to where they can access the electronic version.

An employee handbook helps ensure effective communication with employees about the medical practice's policies, procedures, benefits while outlining the employee's responsibilities from the beginning of employment. It can also be an important compendium of code-of-conduct best practices and employee resources, from dress code to issues of compensation, training and performance management. Workable, a recruiting software, provides an online template and a useful overview for smaller practices building a new employee handbook.[16]

Employee handbooks serve the following functions:

- Serves as a tool for communicating with employees
- Allows the medical practice to state its goals and values
- Provides an opportunity to promote the medical practice's history and accomplishments
- Helps employees understand and follow established rules and expectations
- Enhances the onboarding process
- Ensures that all employees receive the same information and that this information is easily accessible

Employee handbooks can sometimes be considered evidence in a lawsuit; therefore, it is important to have the legal counsel review the handbook both before it is initially distributed to employees and annually, especially as updates are made. Legal areas of concern for handbooks include but are not limited to:

- Introductory and employment-at-will statements
- Overly detailed disciplinary policies
- Non-discrimination and non-harassment policies
- Drug- and violence-free workplace policies
- Manner and frequency of updating and reviewing the handbook

An employee handbook must never represent an enforceable employment contract by including language that appears to constitute an offer that the employee "accepted." To avoid this legal pitfall, include an employment-at-will statement that the attorney has approved. In addition, an employee handbook should have an Acknowledgment of Receipt form that all employees must sign upon receipt of the handbook. Sometimes this form states that the employee has been informed of where to access the electronic version of the handbook and that it is the employee's responsibility to familiarize themselves with its contents. Indeed suggests the receipt be completed on practice letterhead and provide specifics on the issuing party, the person receiving the document and clear indications of its purpose.[17]

Ideally, the medical practice should update and review its employee handbook annually and should include a legal review by the medical practice's attorney. Additionally, every state has slightly different employment laws and regulations that must be considered when developing an employee handbook. Ensure that after the handbook is redistributed to employees, there is a plan in place for re-attestation, so the employees acknowledge receipt of revised policies. It is often helpful to provide a summary of changed sections, so employees know the specifically changed sections, especially for substantial alterations.

Introductions

The aspects of orientation include an introduction of the new employee to their physical workspace and any equipment needed to perform the job adequately. This should include IT equipment, such as computers, information about login and other means of access to the practice's systems. Additionally, any phones or other types of communication devices should be set up and explained if needed.

Along with the physical aspects of the new position, the employee should be introduced to all staff, especially to the manager and the employee's intersection with that individual. During this exercise, any organizational expectations should be laid out and an organizational chart should be provided. Many practices have new employee expectations and these should be spelled out as well.

Functions and Standards

The second part of the orientation concerns information about essential functions and standards of performance. Generally, the immediate supervisor facilitates this departmental orientation to introduce new employees to their job duties and responsibilities and the department's goals, performance standards and policies. This orientation also familiarizes employees with the work area, coworkers and rules. The supervisor should follow up the orientation with effective, consistent communication with the employee, which should include making the employee feel welcomed and relaxed by receiving a greeting each morning and by encouraging questions. An assigned mentor can help facilitate this process.

Pay and Time Management

The pay and time processes should be addressed and carefully explained in the orientation process. Discuss the pay periods, method of how the pay is dispersed and the agreed upon benefits that the practice provides. All employees might not be offered the same benefits; therefore, the benefits for this new team member should be clearly defined.

Remember that orientation can also be a lot of information and new faces for a new employee to absorb at once, so consider breaking orientation sessions into shorter sections. "The last thing you want is an orientation that overwhelms, rather than excites new hires," according to Forbes. "That's why it's a good idea to split orientation sessions over several days, incorporate plenty of breaks and divide extensive topics into digestible chunks of information. Not only does this reduce disruption, but it also gives your new employees the chance to absorb each set of information and recharge before the next section."[18]

New employee orientation and onboarding programs are conducted to familiarize employees with the practice and its culture, reduce turnover and improve the speed at which new employees can perform their roles without oversight. These programs help employees to learn more about their assigned positions, discuss necessary job skills for effective job performance, understand safety and security policies and learn about practice values and the organizational structure. Practices should encourage new employees to ask any questions during the orientation, so they better understand all guidelines that affect and govern their employment relationship. In some cases, individual departments may also conduct orientation programs for specific job duties, responsibilities, expectations and departmental policies and procedures.

5.7 The First 90 Days

The first 90 days of employment should involve careful monitoring of the employee's progress in fulfilling duties. This step is crucial since a medical practice involves patient care or contact. An organized process of review should be implemented. The HR department can employ the following practices for oversight of the new employee's first 90 days in their new role.

- Employing a "buddy system"
- Gathering data from the employee's supervisor
- One-on-one chats with the employee concerning their initial experience
- Acknowledging recognized skills
- Reviewing job roles and responsibilities
- Possible retraining

To reinforce the practice's commitment to its employees, the HR department or administrator should consistently follow up with each new employee during the first 90 days of employment to see if there is a need for more information and/or training. A well-planned, 90-day program provides two important pieces of information—keeping the employee on target and learning about their initial experience—and it is a valuable retention practice.

5.8 Annual Review

Onboarding programs that include mentoring and coaching are more comprehensive and help to ensure a successful transition into the practice. HR follow-up initiatives should include:

- Annual review
- Any needed ongoing training
- Planning for ongoing performance management—this exercise can include a quarterly or semi-annual discussion with the employee. It is useful for the employee to document all instances of their perception concerning their performance, including goals, goals that have been met and future goals.

This conversation with HR or the employee's supervisor should discuss each of these items to help the employee set future goals and ask them to evaluate themselves during this process. These discussions are important and informative for both the new team member and the supervisor or HR person. It might be useful to provide a review chart for the employee to fill out on their perceptions of their performance. Decisions concerning any needed ongoing training and additions to the employee's duties can be decided and discussed at this time. Such practices encourage employee self-awareness and help individuals see themselves as a part of the team and where they fit into the team's goals while helping maintain the practice's vision.

Each aspect of these reviews adds essential information to the annual review, and it is important to understand that these practices should be designed to be results oriented. Notably, a practice might provide opportunities for self-recognition during a significant initiative or other events. Formal reviews need not be the only time reviews are conducted since instances such as those mentioned above provide the opportunity for employee readjustment. Employees want and appreciate feedback. This is a way to develop open communication between new employees and their supervisors.

5.9 Practice in Action

Rapid acquisition and organic growth for a large multispecialty group overwhelmed the onboarding infrastructure of the organization. It resulted in not only an unsatisfactory provider onboarding experience, but also incomplete or inaccurate information being communicated to new members of the team. It became obvious that there was a need to refine and restructure the onboarding process to engage new providers with the larger organization as well as ensure consistent and accurate information was received by those entering the group.

As part of an onboarding restructuring effort, a subgroup was tasked with creating a method, activity or event with the goal of aligning new provider expectations with the organizational culture while ensuring consistent and accurate information delivery. A comprehensive, monthly, half day new provider orientation session was developed and successfully executed that introduced practice processes, thinking, strategies and concepts while creating multiple interpersonal connecting points to thought leaders, subject matter experts and executives. The project is considered successful as the sessions and information presented have been well received by attendees and have met or exceeded goals and objectives of the organization.[19]

5.10 Summary

An employee's introduction to the healthcare workplace, their responsibilities and their team is an important tool in helping to build a long-term relationship. By making strategic choices during the interview process and then following up with a comprehensive onboarding program, HR professionals can help reduce turnover and create more productive and satisfied employees.

Key points discussed in this chapter include:

- HR departments should strive to follow a consistent system for the hiring processes of pre-employment, interviewing and onboarding to ensure all essential tasks are addressed with each new hire to make all go smoothly.

- Medical practices can ensure sound employee selection procedures and avoid unlawful discrimination by carefully developing job-related position descriptions that stick to only duties and required skills for each position. Although an organization should aim to have a diverse candidate pool, identifiers like race, gender, sexual orientation, disability, age and national origin should not be part of the interview process.
- Effective interviewing involves building comfortable communication, managing the direction and flow of the interview, learning about the interviewee's career goals, opening opportunities for questions and active listening.
- Onboarding and new hire orientation brings new employees into the organization by providing information, training, mentoring and coaching during their first 6-12 months of employment. An effective onboarding program should fulfill the promises made during the hiring process and lay the foundation for long-term engagement and performance.
- Annual reviews should discuss planning for ongoing performance management while allowing the employee to set future goals and evaluate themselves.

In the next chapter, we will examine further on-the-job efforts to help retain staff, including development and performance management efforts, as well as the importance of succession planning. We will also discuss proactive strategies during separation.

Notes

1. Gallup. https://www.gallup.com/workplace/398306/quiet-quitting-real.aspx
2. NXT Thing. https://www.nxtthingrpo.com/blog-2022-job-seeker-nation-report/
3. SHRM. https://www.shrm.org/resourcesandtools/tools-and-samples/hr-glossary/pages/human-resource-management-system-hrms.aspx
4. GMS. https://www.groupmgmt.com/blog/post/the-ultimate-guide-to-the-pre-employment-screening-process/
5. U.S. Equal Employment Opportunity Commission. https://www.eeoc.gov/statutes/title-vii-civil-rights-act-1964

6. The Hartford. https://www.thehartford.com/business-insurance/strategy/hiring-first-employee/conduct-interviews

7. Indeed. https://www.indeed.com/hire/c/info/how-to-conduct-a-job-interview

8. Resume Lab. https://resumelab.com/resume/lying

9. GoodHire. https://www.goodhire.com/resources/articles/how-to-do-a-background-check-for-employment/

10. SThree. https://www.sthree.com/en-gb/glossary/o/onboarding/

11. Gallup. https://www.gallup.com/workplace/353096/practical-tips-leaders-better-onboarding-process.aspx

12. SHRM. https://www.shrm.org/resourcesandtools/hr-topics/talent-acquisition/pages/onboarding-key-retaining-engaging-talent.aspx

13. HBR. https://hbr.org/2022/04/onboarding-can-make-or-break-a-new-hires-experience

14. Think Learning. https://www.think-learning.com/onboarding/benefits-of-onboarding/

15. AIHR. https://www.aihr.com/blog/new-employee-orientation/

16. Workable. https://resources.workable.com/employee-handbook-policies

17. Indeed. https://www.indeed.com/hire/c/info/acknowledgement-receipt

18. Forbes. https://www.forbes.com/advisor/business/new-hire-orientation/

19. MGMA. https://www.mgma.com/MGMA/media/files/fellowship%20papers/2018%20Fellows%20Papers/Organizational-Culture-Alignment-Enhanced_FINAL.pdf?ext=.pdf

Chapter 6

Employee Development, Performance Management and Separation

6.1 Autonomy, Mastery and Purpose

This chapter will examine how the use of performance reviews, employee recognition and a variety of career growth opportunities can help improve employee engagement and strengthen retention within a practice. As a part of the longer employee lifecycle, we will also examine strategies relating to succession planning, to keep a practice fully functional as managers or key staff step down, as well as some best practices regarding succession planning and separation.

Autonomy is defined as the freedom to act. According to NIH, job autonomy in the workplace involves employees' control and decisions over work methods, work arrangements and work standards, which differs from simple freedom, in that it gives employees the opportunity to make decisions at work and to have a voice in what they do.[1] Lack of autonomy is caused by any challenge an employee may face that stops them from acting freely to complete their role.

This frustration is the largest detractor from employee engagement, yet challenges in medical groups are often pushed aside as systemically impossible to change. The strategic HR leader must reach past the normal confines of the functional role to be a business leader and reasonably guide operations to address challenges head-on. Not doing so will continue to affect employee engagement negatively, and any survey measuring engagement will continue to demonstrate a lack of attention to resolving core issues fundamental to employee autonomy.

Some good leaders may muse that full autonomy of all staff members will lead to individual interpretations of right and wrong, therefore efficiency, scalability and group focus on strategic outcomes will be impossible. The trick of both HR and operational leadership is to find the balance of guideposts within which staff at all levels and performing all roles can simultaneously feel autonomous to complete the tasks of each day without constant impingement on their judgment, but still offer guidance that directs those decisions in the right way for the betterment of the medical group.

Natural tension is the source of a constant hum of conflict. When managed well in medical groups, productive conflict is the foundation for difficult-but-effective decision making. When left unmanaged, this naturally occurring conflict between professional autonomy and organizational direction can derail staff, causing bad patient experiences and outcomes while fostering a very unhealthy work environment.

Human Motivation

In 2009, Daniel Pink published a seminal book on human motivation called *Drive: The Surprising Truth About What Motivates Us*.[2] To debunk outdated theories of human motivation, Pink defines three modern elements of human motivation now that our workforce has moved away from labor with mechanical steps resulting in a single direction: Pink describes these as:

- **Autonomy:** ability to self-govern and make uncoerced decisions
- **Mastery:** comprehensive knowledge or skill
- **Purpose:** end goal or essential function

Medical group employees are expected to make decisions, use creativity to solve problems and engage in higher-level thinking to serve patients and families in novel ways. But compensation is not a motivator once reasonable compensation is mutually agreed upon between the employee and employer.

Pink argues for an update from the old-fashioned culture of reward and punishment found in most businesses to a more self-directed model of motivation. According to Mind Tools, while autonomy motivates employees to think creatively, mastery is the desire to improve, which is appealing to employees who believe that their potential is unlimited.[3] Encouraging employees to find purpose in their work will help them stay hard-working, productive and engaged, while connecting their personal goals to organizational targets. Combined, these three levers can be used by employers to drive higher levels of performance in employees.

Strategic HR practices like performance management, training, leadership development, succession planning, retention and recognition programs as well as engagement surveys are all tools that help organizations measure and improve these three core concepts of autonomy, mastery and purpose. These strategic HR practices are sound and necessary but fall short when they lose alignment with the core motivational concepts that employers want to build with employees. According to SolveHR, the HR function has lost credibility when the completion of transactional HR processes is disconnected from the desired strategic results of employee motivation and performance.[4] As medical groups choose to deploy versions of these tools and concepts, variability in the chosen process is less critical if the desired end goal is ensured.

Leadership Development Disconnect

Susan Aloi, PhD, FACMPE, found that there can be a disconnect in leadership development at practices. "In all of my research over the past 24 months," Aloi told MGMA in 2023, "I found that 80% of health systems believed … the investment in leadership development is a strategic imperative, [yet] only 20% of them actually invest in leadership development."[5]

Aloi pointed to five common barriers cited by healthcare organization leaders for not investing in leadership development:

1. **The lack of financial and staff resources** stands out as a primary deterrent, preventing many organizations from committing to leadership development. Concerns about expenses and resource limitations hinder the creation of the necessary infrastructure for these programs.

2. **Short-term focus** emerges as another roadblock, as organizations prioritize immediate results over long-term development. The pressure to meet financial targets often overshadows the importance of building a strong leadership team capable of navigating future challenges. This short-sighted approach may hamper growth and hinder organizations from achieving their full potential.

3. **A lack of understanding** also plagues some organizations, as they fail to grasp the critical nature of developing leaders. Perceiving it as an unnecessary expense rather than a vital investment, they overlook the long-term benefits such development programs offer.

4. **Resistance to change** further exacerbates the situation, with leaders hesitant to invest in developing new leaders who may challenge their authority and disrupt the status quo.

5. **Lack of time to develop their leaders**. Building effective leaders is a time-consuming process that demands careful attention and investment. However, the reluctance to commit these resources hampers the growth and potential of leaders and the organization.

6.2 Engagement and Retention Strategies

Groups' standard HR processes to manage employee performance include several exercises and processes, including reviews, retention interviews and recognition programs. All of these processes and their permutations can help a leadership team engage employees in constructive conversations about how to improve their autonomy of role, thus improving their motivation to perform that role to the best of their ability. A role review, for both long-tenured and new employees, will bring to light both major and minor issues.

Likely, that same employee might need help understanding the challenge of fixing the issues but has ideas for improving their own life. The role review is the conduit to uncover the issues, discuss possible solutions and then set the next steps to improve the employee's challenges. The role review as an HR process will not solve the issues but is a proactive vehicle to bring solutions to the table for evaluation and resolution.

A skills gap analysis is a helpful tool to identify the skills that employees need but lack to carry out responsibilities of their role. It not only provides opportunities to boost individual learning and development, but it can also help HR professionals gain insights for strategic workforce planning that can improve recruitment efforts to gain a competitive edge.[6]

Retention or stay interviews are similar conversations with a slightly different twist to getting at the heart of an employee's issue—not necessarily tied to their role—and what that employee appreciates about their workplace. All of this serves as valuable methods for engagement and retention. According to a 2022 survey from Paychex, a payroll and HR solutions platform, more than one-quarter of HR decision makers polled say they use stay interviews to help increase retention.[7]

Retention Surveys and Reviews

Suppose a team member proves promising and shows themselves as a valuable practice member. In that case, it should be an early undertaking of the HR team to conduct a retention interview. A worst-case scenario is promising employees engaging in job searches when the practice has essentially invested time and resources in their training, not to mention the unpleasant task of beginning again after the investment has been made for this hire. Such surveys are valuable as treasure hunts for employees' thoughts on job satisfaction.

Exhibit 6.1 Retention Survey Question Guidelines

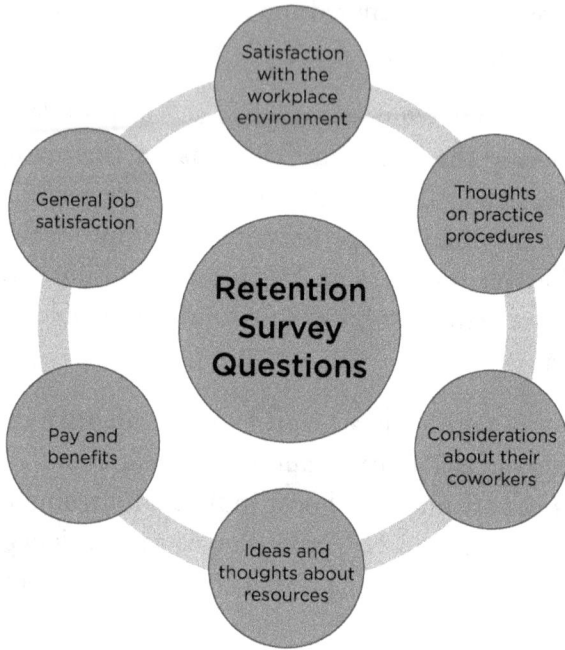

By asking the right questions, the survey can be key in improving the employee experience and increasing your organization's retention rate. Conducting this survey provides opportunities to boost employee engagement, uncover skills gaps and decrease absenteeism.

This list is not exhaustive by any means, but HR leaders can craft the survey that best fits the vision and outreach. Some questions are general, but some should be specific to the practice's needs and its leadership.

Employee Recognition

Recognition is the affirmation of autonomous behavior that finds the ideal path between the strategic guideposts of the organization. There are countless recognition programs, (some that have already been discussed elsewhere in this book) all of which contribute to employee satisfaction and have a place inside a medical group—large and small—but dependent on the recognition recipient's preference. Public or group recognition is powerful, as is a single email thanking an employee for a specific job well done. Be targeted in the recognition provided to the employee—what did they do well so they can continue to do it? Recognizing and rewarding positive and exceptional behavior reinforces that the behavior and action are highly desired in the organization and encouraged to repeat. According to Indeed, these run the gamut from traditional "years of service" awards to employee appreciation events, as well as monetary rewards and acknowledgments on social media.[8] Rewards and recognition help employees identify that their organization values them and their contributions to the team's success. When employees are recognized, they feel seen—they are positively contributing to the culture in a way that elevates the experience for both patients and the community. This creates a feeling of well-being for individual performance and promotes retention within the organization.

Establishing a framework or a set of options for regular recognition within the practice is a critical action for the strategic HR leader. Dictating a group-wide recognition program will force the issue for a time but will feel inauthentic for some and, therefore, will be short-lived. Finding various ways to identify and recognize excellent contributions is the key to long-lasting employee motivation because their autonomous decisions are recognized as excellent.

Rewards tied to recognition are equally broad in variety and purpose. Be careful to distinguish best pay practices for the total rewards program from rewards tied to spot recognition. Many groups avoid cash bonuses in rewards programs to create a clear delineation between spot rewards tied to recognition, differentially from a quarterly or year-end bonus tied to goal performance. According to Bamboo HR, more than one-third of employees surveyed said they would rather be recognized for their accomplishments in a company-wide email from an executive than receive a $500 bonus that wasn't openly publicized.[9]

Each group's culture of rewards and recognition is different. Creating the parameters, communicating the rules of engagement in rewards programs, and providing clear and consistent feedback is vital for a productive practice. This provides a clear sense of direction, informing the employee if they are heading down the correct path. Two-way communication also provides essential data to leaders to determine if their employees' needs are being met. Leaders can significantly affect the working relationship and the employee's engagement by:

- Fostering work-life balance
- Fostering professional development and advancement opportunities
- Connecting the employees' idea of meaningful work to the mission, vision, purpose

As the employees' needs and expectations shift with time, their stance and preferences are generally consistent with the market and personal circumstances.

6.3 Intersection of Role, Manager and Organizational Expectations with New Hires

Each element of the employee value proposition has a coinciding employer value. The strategic HR leader must clearly articulate each of those employer benefits—and communicating those benefits to other leaders and staff at the right time is equally important. According to Justin Holland, CEO and co-founder of HealthJoy, the more communication the better, especially when it comes to focusing on the value of those benefits, soliciting regular feedback on benefits and even learning how employees like to get info on their benefits—namely their mobile devices.[10]

When strategically planning quarterly review points, you can steer the next quarter's focus by picking out the areas where the group is performing well or underperforming on expected value elements. Daily or weekly team huddles can help reinforce and recognize how the group experiences employee value while discussing how it benefits the group and its patients. Suppose employee selection in the hiring process puts equal emphasis on each element. In the case of behavioral interviewing, answers that address the importance and adherence to organizational culture and teamwork become equally important to pay and opportunities. If candidates ask about how the work environment deals with prompt pay along with opportunities for higher earnings and career progression, then it's clear that these will be the core values of the potential new staff. Suppose another candidate asks questions about who they'll be working with, how they could leverage a mentor relationship at the practice, or what the group does together for fun during and after hours. In any case, it'll be clear what the candidates value.

Therefore, employers need to articulate for each employee—new or long-tenured—how their medical group balances each element of the value proposition to deliver the most value for the medical group. Showing employees what the medical group needs from employees to be successful can be a win-win and eye-opening conversation between employer and employee. Transparently discussing how patient visits earn medical revenue, which in turn pays for staff salaries, easily explains why showing up on time for a shift or rooming a patient quickly means success for both the practice and the employee. Showing a new hire a picture of the end-to-end patient visit experience and all the handoffs between different staff members is an easier way to describe why good teamwork and positive staff relationships are critical to making the work of the group not only efficient but more enjoyable.

6.4 Performance Management

All employees want to know what a job well done looks like and receive consistent feedback to deliver on that expectation. Performance management is simply a tool to produce alignment, create continuous improvement and ensure each employee is focused on the priorities that will most benefit the organization in its pursuit of strategic outcomes. This encourages each team member to focus on their results and accomplishments—not just activities and the swirl of the busy day-to-day world—that lead them to perform excellently.

According to AIHR, performance management is a set of processes and systems aimed at developing employees so they perform their job to the best of their ability.[11] That allows employees to reach their potential and boost their success, while also meeting the practice's strategic goals.

123

An effective performance management process consists of a few key elements that provide a roadmap to an employee's future in the organization.

Exhibit 6.2 Key Elements of Effective Performance Management

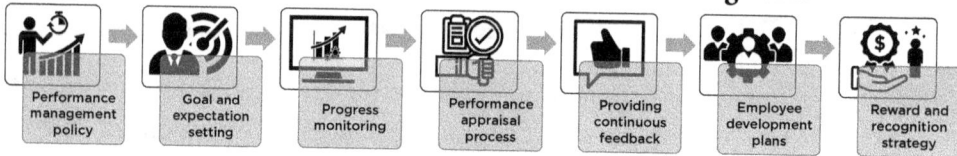

| Performance management policy | Goal and expectation setting | Progress monitoring | Performance appraisal process | Providing continuous feedback | Employee development plans | Reward and recognition strategy |

The words "performance appraisal" or "annual review" can generate nervous anticipation, excitement, dread or, worst of all, time wasting. Because things happen quickly in medical practices, it's more important than ever to modernize performance management practices for better agility. Annual performance is erratic—an employee has a strong week of performance and then comes to work late for two of the following three shifts. In a single month, an employee could be both a strong performer worthy of reward, recognition, and growth while also being a performance problem whose ability to perform their role with trust and expertise is questionable. An annual evaluation of that example employee could be inconclusive at best.

Be more agile to match the pace and demands of the ever-shifting healthcare regulatory environment and the patients served. Performance management should be organic, meaning it seizes the moments as they arise. Finding opportunities for positive feedback on a job well done, coupled with constructive feedback in areas needing improvement, sets employees up for success. The sooner you get started, the sooner they can succeed. According to MIT HR, it's important to structure the review to offer shared responsibility in a collaborative and open feedback process, making a commitment to continuous improvement and follow-through as a result of the review.[12]

Coaching

Coaching skills are crucial for people managers and are the key to developing employees that meet the ever-demanding needs of the healthcare regulatory environment. It's finding paths to empower employees to perform consistently and at increasingly higher levels. Exceptional coaches challenge their teams and do not accept the status quo. Coaching creates an environment of accountability, builds trust and open communications, and ultimately increases productivity because employees know the goals and how to achieve them. Providing coaching and feedback once a year or expecting that someone's performance will improve with one touchpoint is unrealistic.

Exhibit 6.3 Coaching vs. Mentoring Chart

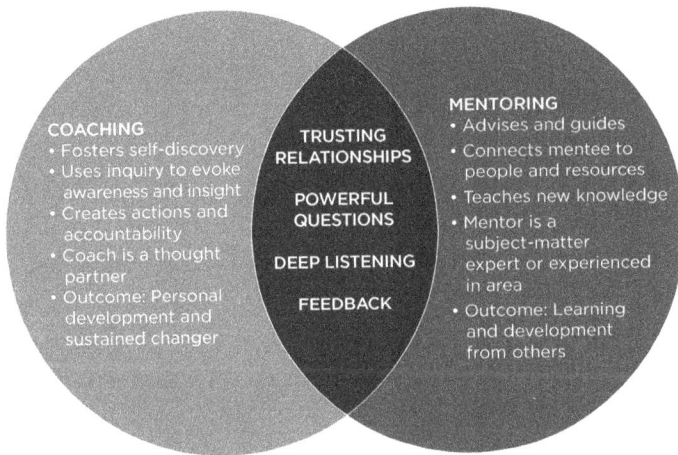

COACHING
• Fosters self-discovery
• Uses inquiry to evoke awareness and insight
• Creates actions and accountability
• Coach is a thought partner
• Outcome: Personal development and sustained changer

TRUSTING RELATIONSHIPS

POWERFUL QUESTIONS

DEEP LISTENING

FEEDBACK

MENTORING
• Advises and guides
• Connects mentee to people and resources
• Teaches new knowledge
• Mentor is a subject-matter expert or experienced in area
• Outcome: Learning and development from others

Sample Coaching Dialogue

An MGMA article from 2021 shares a few distinctions between a coach and a mentor: "A coach asks powerful questions, rather than giving advice as a mentor might do, to stimulate critical thinking, prompt self-reflection and generate action steps toward a defined outcome. A coach does not need to be a SME in the topic of the conversation, but rather skilled in the process of evoking insight and generating committed actions by the coachee."[13]

In the following exchange from the article, the coach asks powerful questions to promote self-discovery. The coach listens and mirrors what he or she is hearing, observing and sensing to bring awareness to the "coachee." In concluding, the coach builds in commitment and accountability to ensure forward movement.

- **Coach:** How are you today?
- **Coachee:** Okay. A lot of changes are going on. Most of my team and I are now working from home. The staff have been working long hours to cover the staffing shortage that has resulted due to COVID.
- **Coach:** Based upon the tone of your voice, it sounds like it has been challenging.
- **Coachee:** Yes, this is a dedicated team who continuously goes above and beyond to support patients and their team. I want to support them but I'm not sure of the best way.
- **Coach:** What about this situation is weighing most on you?
- **Coachee:** I think it is part of my leadership responsibility to be there for them and help them where needed. I have seen staff more frustrated than before. One person raised their voice to another during a meeting yesterday and that has not happened before. I am concerned about the well-being of staff.
- **Coach:** I can tell you care about your team. It sounds like you have also been impacted.
- **Coachee:** This is something I have also had to work on given my husband and kids are also home. It's hard staying connected with staff. I have had to consciously ... [talks about actions she has taken to work through this transition ... and is still working on it]. This is reminding me that we are all in this together. I am wondering if I should have an open conversation with my team about well-being, even sharing some of my own challenges and talking about how we can support each other.
- **Coach:** That sounds like a healthy approach for you and your team. What is a step that will help you move in that direction?
- **Coachee:** We have a team meeting tomorrow. There is time on the agenda so I think I will raise the issue and see what kind of response I get.

- • **Coach:** So, you are going to talk with your team tomorrow. Would you let me know how it goes after the meeting?

Setting Goals

Just as it is essential for an organization to have a strategy and a road map, employees need to create a road map to set themselves up for success and provide their manager with a clear objective to coach them and reach their goals. An excellent way to ensure that the sense of direction and organization of milestones is in place is by utilizing SMART goals (Specific, Measurable, Achievable, Realistic and Time-bound) – allowing managers to more effectively set and benchmark their goal-setting process.[14] Many organizations build this into their existing performance management plans/reviews and recurring one-on-one meetings between new hires and their managers.

Exhibit 6.4 SMART Goals

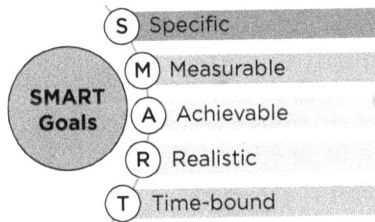

SMART goals stem from an organization's strategy, directly or indirectly, counting each employee's goals in the expected outcomes for their performance. Suppose someone's goal is to consistently room every patient within ten minutes of check-in each day and week. In that case, it only has meaning if connected to an overarching strategy of the positive patient experience.

Identify Barriers to Goals

A frequently overlooked component of goal setting is the realistic discussion about barriers or obstacles that will stand in the way of an individual reaching a goal. There can be various instances that can take an employee off their SMART goal roadmap, but generally these barriers involve the following:[15]

- Lack of alignment
- Lack of feedback
- Lack of resources
- Lack of commitment
- Lack of flexibility

Realism in the goal-setting process sets the employee up for success and creates realistic expectations for outcome achievement for the manager. Early identification of barriers can also lead to resolving those challenges, allowing for even more significant achievement by the employee during the goal's time period. Finally, the identification of barriers that shape realistic goals allows managers to avoid contentious negative performance conversations downstream if poor goal achievement cannot be blamed on barriers outside an employee's control.

6.5 Succession Planning

Succession management is a strategic process and mindset designed to ensure that a robust talent pipeline is ready for future leadership roles. A well-designed succession process creates a competitive edge for the organization and mitigates the risk of not having well-prepared leaders to assume critical leadership roles. Succession planning has a viable place in any strategically-run medical practice. But, according to an MGMA Conference Board survey, developing the next generation of leaders is still a lower priority for many healthcare CEOs.[16] In essence, succession planning begins the funneling process of nurturing talent by training such talent for future management roles. This process encourages team members to look ahead, set goals and see themselves in future leadership roles. Learning and growing should always be an integral part of the medical practice and supervisors should be tasked with looking for talent who would be good candidates for an upwardly mobile process. Maintaining a list of such team members will help the process.

An example of this concept would be where a team member who is a talented medical assistant who shows a solid ability to make patients feel comfortable as they do patient intake before the patient sees the physician. This employee's tone, patient relationships and gift of accuracy that instills comfort (often in anxious patients) sets a good atmosphere for the physician when they meet with the patient. This medical assistant has also indicated that they would like to receive more training. He or she might fill a future position or specialize in working with an incoming doctor's practice requiring specific medical knowledge. The supervisor takes note of this and considers them a viable candidate for the coordination of the group of medical assistants. The name is forwarded for the possibility of further training and an upcoming opening for the coordinator position.

Such a scenario shows the way a well-managed medical practice can function. Any practice has a turnover for a variety of reasons. Keeping a list of potential candidates for these positions creates a good practice for talent management and encourages less disruption in the practice. Now they can begin training for the position before it is vacated.

Promotion, Moving Roles/Transfers, Knowledge and Institutional Transfer

A form of promotion and the possible methods of identifying individuals who can fill future positions is addressed above. Promotions and transfers are ongoing in any medical practice, and promotions and transfers are often necessary. Promotions and transfers can occur for various reasons, such as management-mandated, employee requests, and fluctuations in the need for team members in various areas of the practice. Additionally, a promotion based on a history of good performance or signaling from the employee that learning more or moving to another team in the practice can be another reason for transfer or promotion.

Transfer can happen when an employee has difficulties performing a job or has issues with other team members. Supervisors must be careful to know how the various team members are functioning, their wishes and how they appear suitable to their daily tasks. Meetings among the supervisors can be held where information on team members is discussed. Careful notes should be kept in such meetings and federal laws of employment, such as laws governing disabilities or discrimination, must be considered and applied.

A transfer and promotion policy is essential, and it should be carefully carried out as written. This comes into play when multiple employees are qualified for a position or management requires a transfer for staffing considerations. But promotions must be awarded based on good job performance that has been carefully documented.

6.6 Cultural Impact on Separation

Employment separation is the process where an employee separates from employment for various reasons and actions. Times will occur when employment must terminate and the working relationship between employee and employer discontinues. The policy of the various termination situations should be clearly spelled out to employees early in the hiring process. This is one of the most important roles of the HR team. The HR policies concerning work separation should be clearly and completely delineated in the employee handbook, including the various reasons for separation. Such things include voluntary separation, involuntary separation, the applicable laws and the processes for ending the employment relationship with the medical practice.

Communication Regarding Separation

Regardless of the reason, termination is a disruption to the practice. It affects many levels of the work area, from management down to many of the team that works with the terminated individual. When a termination occurs, one of the first activities should be to hold meetings with the remaining staff. "If you have a small team, let everyone know at once," according to the U.S. Chamber of Commerce. "Regardless of when and how you notify the rest of your team, make sure your employees know who they can talk to if they have any questions or concerns, and ensure the messaging is respectful and straightforward."[17] These team members shoulder the effect of the reduction in staff. Handled carefully, this action should help with undercurrents of gossip, questioning and fear the remaining staff might experience. Open communication is essential since it helps these employees to understand that the practice will continue as usual and that the employee's place in the practice remains important.

However, during these meetings, nothing about the particulars should be discussed and privacy must be carefully maintained. The exit process should be carefully orchestrated according to the Employee handbook and in compliance with federal and state laws. All aspects of the exit process must be made clear to the employee, along with the reasons for the termination. All of this should happen under the umbrella of prior employee performance management sessions that include coaching and discussions of ways performance could be improved. Throughout each of the exit processes discussed below, careful documentation is a must. All interactions should be diligently recorded.

Voluntary Separation

Several forms of voluntary separation exist. These include but are not limited to:

- Retirement
- Leaving for other employment
- A disgruntled employee quitting

As an employee leaves a practice, the practice managers have expectations that the employee should meet. Proper notice, as spelled out in the Employee Handbook, should be given and a letter of resignation should be delivered to the HR manager. An exit interview with the employee should be conducted where information about leaving the practice is given.

Involuntary Separation

Practices experience involuntary separations for myriad reasons: layoffs, down/right-sizing, mergers and acquisitions, practice failure and furloughs. Layoffs are likely an unpleasant event for any practice, depending on the number of staff involved. They often involve employees who might be performing well, but the practice finds it necessary to reduce staff numbers for the reasons mentioned above.

Termination

Termination occurs when an employee fails to perform duties or assignments properly, demonstrates egregious behavior issues, or fails to comply with carefully delineated policies listed in the handbook. "In the case of an involuntary termination, an exit interview is not only an opportunity to tell the employee that their employment is ending, but also to provide them with a clear and precise explanation of the reason(s) why," notes attorney Missy Oakley, with Barran Liebman LLP.[18] The reason(s) for the termination must be carefully articulated to the exiting employee. A termination letter should be considered wherein the reasons for the termination are documented. It is important to conduct a termination or "exit" interview and to avoid common pitfalls, such as high emotions, arguing, using platitudes and creating any personal atmosphere, in case the HR manager feels some emotional involvement.

Professionalism is a key component of the termination process. The processes surrounding separation, both voluntary and involuntary, must be handled with clarity, careful adherence to the federal and state laws, and carefully delineated definitions concerning what each of the actions and processes means to the employee, as well as the stated methods discussed in the Employee Manual. All steps of the termination process must be documented, including the interactions with the employee and the HR individual conducting the action. It is imperative that the documentation is detailed and clearly stated. The impetus to carefully handle and document this process is straightforward; disgruntled separating employees can create a fraught atmosphere within the practice and after separation occurs. Emotions are high, and individuals can become defensive, difficult and damaging. It is important to make the termination discussion as respectful as possible. The person should be treated fairly and with dignity. The terminated employee will still be representing your employer brand. Preserve the brand as much as possible.

At-Will Separation

Terminating an "at-will" employment refers to the ability of both the employer and the employee to end the employment relationship at any time, for any reason, as long as the reason for termination is not illegal.

However, there are certain limitations and exceptions to consider when terminating an employee in an at-will employment arrangement.[19]

While employers have the right to terminate an at-will employee, they cannot do so for illegal reasons. Discrimination based on race, sex, age (40 and over), nation of origin, disability, or genetic information is prohibited.

Exceptions to At-Will Employment include:

- Public Policy: Some states have exceptions based on public policy. For example, terminating an employee for filing a workers' compensation claim may be prohibited in certain states.
- Express or Implied Contracts: In some states, policies described in an employee handbook may be considered implied contracts, and termination must adhere to those policies.
- Good Faith: In certain states, employers may be required to have just cause for termination or may be prohibited from terminating employees for reasons motivated by malice or made in bad faith.

When dealing with at-will employment, taking legal considerations into account is important. By consulting an attorney and documenting reasons for termination with justifiable causes, employers can protect themselves from litigation due to retaliation and discrimination claims.

Severance Packages

In the event of a layoff, severance packages may be offered. Severance packages depend on each situation and the circumstances of the company's decision. If the employee is involuntarily separated and has done well as a team member, the practice may offer a severance package that provides compensation after termination of employment. Such packages are often referred to as a separation agreement since they often entail legal separation agreements. Severance packages should be discussed in the employee manual and stand as a legal agreement that protects the practice from lawsuits involving possible wrongful dismissal.

Severance packages can offer a variety of compensations:

- Use of accrued PTO, vacation or holiday time
- More payment that reflects the months of the employee's service
- Additions to retirement accounts
- Possible stock options
- Possible help with locating new work

In the case of layoffs or voluntary termination, employees may require a confidentiality agreement or guarantee that the exiting employee will not work for competitors. Such can be the case if a practice works with specialized care or holds patents on some specific treatments. Reference local laws regarding non-compete clauses. Some cities and states prohibit non-compete clauses. The non-compete clause cannot prevent the terminated employee from working in their profession. Consider also that organizations such as the AMA have been active in attempting to ban many physician non-compete provisions.[20]

Within medical groups, it is reasonable to anticipate tension or outright confrontation between staff members, and the repercussions of that environment are transparent and unfortunate. Harmful patient interactions, poor staff morale and an untenable work arrangement mean immediate actions must be taken to minimally correct bad staff behavior or, worse, terminate certain team members for their destructive behavior. But by examining the balance of value being provided to the employees, these situations can be remedied before they even occur.

Conflict

Team conflicts within a medical setting can come from a variety of circumstances. Conflicts can arise from issues such as poor execution of goals and procedures, ethical disputes, role conflicts, or misallocating practice resources. These problems arise from poor job performance or poor training, and each should be remedied during performance management, in further training or a correction of inadequate training. According to the American Nurses Association, some practical tips for navigating conflict include:[21]

- Foster open communication
- Mediate and negotiate
- Identify underlying issues
- Encourage empathy
- Seek a compromise
- Provide guidance and coaching
- Encourage professional behavior
- Follow established policies and procedures

Team issues such as jealousy or personality conflicts can also arise from emotional issues. In instances such as these, conflict resolution can come into play. Frustration and unhappiness come from missed expectations, and conflict resolution can be of great value in these situations. It is instructive to consider that conflict can be valuable since it can highlight a weakness in the chain of the team's structure and organizational issues that arise. At these times, a good manager can identify the issue and take steps to correct it, strengthening the overall team and the practice's performance.

6.7 Practice in Action

Tony Schirer, Executive Director of Wyoming's Cheyenne OBGYN, says he uses his annual reviews as a stepping stone to help establish training and development goals with his staff, many of whom worked through the entire pandemic period. "We try not to use a one-to-five scale with our open-ended questions. I think where the clarity comes in is allowing them to ask questions. What are the wins we had this year? What are the wins going forward? What do we need to work on? Our evaluations are more like, Are they doing their role? Are they exceeding their role? Are they learning? What can we do to help them improve, what skills do they want to learn? That's where we start to pull out the other piece of what they want to do with their career."

Those open-ended evaluation questions, Shirer says, help begin a conversation that can help establish measurable goals and KPIs. "How can we better engage our teams towards these organizational skills? Over the last few years, it feels like we've been running with our hair on fire, and we haven't had any time to sit down and look seriously at our goals—like improving patient satisfaction scores, or improving our no-call-no-show rates. So we set goals, all the way down to the individual level, and have each employee set up three goals that they can do to help the department, and that helps the organization as well. We find things that we can measure, either quarterly or monthly, and we meet with these individuals quarterly, instead of annually, to see how they are doing on these goals and what they need."

"A little prompting," Schirer says, "can go a long way, as well as the opportunity to earn more. If we see some things that we think that they might do well at, we will encourage them or give them a push to say, 'have you ever thought about pursuing this?' For those that say, 'yes, that is exactly what I'd like to do,' we let them start doing some research on what that really means. For instance, our sonographers are probably the big one, where we always try to evaluate their skills and make sure that they're up to date on the newest technology. The community college here will also put on two-day seminars like crucial conversations, how to be a leader for the first time, conflict management ... so we will send them out and bring back whatever material they learn, and then we get to discuss what is learned to the whole team. I had a front-office staff person who was bilingual in English and Spanish and I encouraged her to become a certified medical translator – we paid for her to do that, and then we utilized those skills here in the clinic. And she also earned a little higher wage because of that tremendous benefit for us. I've also had MAs that we thought would make great RNs. So we at least throw that out, and I've had a couple who have taken advantage of that."

6.8 Summary

From the beginning to the end of the employee lifecycle, HR professionals must work on providing clear, competent and unbiased support for their employees. Frequent and well-communicated programs to foster employees' growth can also help offset the challenges which occur as employees separate from the business.

Key points discussed in this chapter include:

- Autonomy, mastery and purpose are three modern elements that define human motivation. Strategic HR practices like performance management, training, leadership development, succession planning, along with retention and recognition programs can help organizations measure and improve these three core concepts within their staff.

- HR and operational leadership can collaborate to find balanced guideposts that allow staff to feel autonomous in their roles while offering guidance that directs those decisions towards the betterment of the medical group.

- Establishing a framework for regular recognition within the practice is a critical action for the strategic HR leader. Rewards and recognition help employees identify that their organization values them and their contributions to the team's success.

- Performance management that is organic and agile can match the pace and demands of the ever-shifting healthcare regulatory environment as well as the patients served. Through coaching and SMART goal setting, performance management can create continuous organizational improvement.

- A well-designed succession plan not only mitigates the risk of not having well-prepared leaders to assume critical roles, but it can also create a competitive edge for a practice. As turnover remains high, keeping a list of internal candidates for these roles creates a good practice for talent management and encourages less disruption in the practice.

- The processes surrounding separation—both voluntary and involuntary—must be handled with clarity, professionalism and careful adherence to the law. HR policies concerning work separation should be clearly and completely delineated in the employee handbook, including the various reasons for separation.

The next chapter will lay out federal labor laws and discuss best practices for ensuring a compliant and safe organization.

Notes

1. NIH. https://www.ncbi.nlm.nih.gov/pmc/articles/PMC10295641/

2. Daniel Pink. *Drive: The Surprising Truth About What Motivates Us.* https://www.danpink.com/books/drive/

3. Mind Tools. https://www.mindtools.com/asmdp60/pinks-autonomy-mastery-and-purpose-framework

4. SolveHR. https://blog.solvehr.com/transactional-and-strategic-hr-why-you-want-both-in-your-business

5. MGMA. https://www.mgma.com/mgma-stat/is-an-in-house-leadership-development-program-right-for-your-medical-group

6. AIHR. https://www.aihr.com/blog/skills-gap-analysis/

7. SHRM. https://www.shrm.org/hr-today/news/hr-magazine/spring-2023/pages/how-managers-can-use-stay-interviews-to-improve-retention.aspx

8. Indeed. https://www.indeed.com/hire/c/info/employee-recognition-examples

9. Bamboo HR. https://www.bamboohr.com/blog/difference-reward-and-recognition

10. Benefits Pro. https://www.benefitspro.com/2021/07/23/3-keys-to-clear-benefits-communication/

11. AIHR. https://www.aihr.com/blog/what-is-performance-management/

12. MIT HR. https://hr.mit.edu/performance/reviews

13. MGMA. https://www.mgma.com/articles/coaching-and-mentoring-methods-leaders-can-use-to-develop-talent

14. Forbes. https://www.forbes.com/advisor/business/smart-goals/

15. LinkedIn. https://www.linkedin.com/advice/0/what-most-common-roadblocks-achieving-smart

16. MGMA. https://www.mgma.com/articles/succession-management-an-essential-strategy-for-organizational-success

17. U.S. Chamber of Commerce. https://www.uschamber.com/co/run/human-resources/how-to-communicate-employee-termination

18. VA Lawyers Weekly. https://valawyersweekly.com/2023/03/07/employee-termination-best-practices-exit-interviews-and-final-paychecks/

19. SHRM. https://www.shrm.org/topics-tools/news/employee-relations/employment-will-isnt-blank-check-to-terminate-employees-dont-like

20. AMA. https://www.ama-assn.org/medical-residents/transition-resident-attending/ama-backs-effort-ban-many-physician-noncompete

21. ANA. https://www.nursingworld.org/resources/individual/nurse-managers/conflict-resolution-in-nursing/

Chapter 7

Compliance with Labor Laws

7.1 Incorporating Labor Laws into HR strategy

Developing HR strategies that align with business needs and cultural development is vital for any healthcare organization to succeed. As these strategies are developed, they must first comply with up-to-date laws and regulations to protect the organization along with current and prospective employees from such things as occupational hazards, harassment, discrimination, wage and benefit discrepancies, unlawful termination and litigation. Other than avoiding legal repercussions, there are several reasons that motivate organizations to observe labor laws. According to *HR Digest*, three of the most common consequences for non-compliance can involve a loss of resources, loss of talent and instant bad reputation.[1] While there are countless local and state labor laws that also apply, this chapter will focus on some of the main federal laws and governing bodies that must oversee any healthcare organization's HR strategy. In addition, this chapter will cover HR's responsibilities for ensuring a compliant HR strategy and organization overall.

7.2 Workplace Discrimination Laws

EEO

The Equal Employment Opportunity laws protect against discrimination in the workplace and apply to all stages of an employee's lifecycle from pre-hire through termination. These laws are enforced by the Equal Employment Opportunity Commission (EEOC).[2] The EEOC is responsible for enforcing federal laws that make it illegal to discriminate against a job applicant or an employee because of the person's race, color, religion, sex (including pregnancy and related conditions, gender identity, and sexual orientation), national origin, age (40 or older), disability or genetic information. Most employers with at least 15 employees are covered by EEOC laws (20 employees in age discrimination cases). The laws apply to all types of work situations, including hiring, firing, promotions, harassment, training, wages and benefits.[3]

The EEOC has the authority to investigate charges of discrimination against employers and practices who are covered by the law. Their role in an investigation is to fairly and accurately assess the allegations in the charge and then make a finding. There are several laws enforced under the EEOC umbrella including the following:

Title VII

Title VII of the Civil Rights Act of 1964, as amended, protects employees and job applicants from employment discrimination based on race, color, religion, sex and national origin. Title VII protection covers the full spectrum of employment decisions, including recruitment, selections, terminations, and other decisions concerning terms and conditions of employment.[4]

It is important for the medical practice to have clear equal employment opportunity and anti-harassment policies, complaint processes, and conduct audits to identify potential areas of discrimination. Developing an employee complaint policy provides staff with an orderly process to promptly and equitably resolve any concern or complaint.

To ensure a safe and respectful work environment, medical practices can engage in the following:

- Written policy that clearly defines harassment while providing specific reporting methods and corrective measures

- Training that ensures all staff in leadership roles understand their specific responsibilities to report any incidents
- Annual management review of policies and procedures regarding their roles and responsibilities in reporting harassment
- Annual training sessions and a review of policies with staff
- Take every complaint seriously to actively provide a respectful and welcoming practice environment for staff and patients alike
- Research and understand harassment laws at both the state and federal level along with employer liabilities and responsibilities
- Documentation of employees' awareness of written policies along with any training sessions attended, complaints filed, investigative methods/outcomes and corrective actions taken
- Notices posted in prominent places reminding staff of policies

ADA

The Americans with Disabilities Act of 1990 (ADA) makes it unlawful to discriminate in employment against a qualified individual with a disability. The ADA also outlaws discrimination against individuals with disabilities in state and local government services, public accommodations, transportation and telecommunications. State and local civil rights enforcement agencies work with the EEOC to enforce ADA laws.[5]

Medical practices should develop processes for handling accommodation requests, educate leadership on ADA compliance and create an inclusive workplace. Practices must also be informed on who is covered under the ADA, since cases may vary involving applicants and employees as independent contractors are not covered under the law.

Reasonable accommodations under the ADA may include but are not limited to:

- Making facilities readily accessible to and usable by a person with disabilities
- Job restructuring
- Modifying work schedules
- Reassigning the employee to a vacant position
- Acquiring or modifying equipment or devices
- Adjusting or modifying exams/training materials/policies
- Providing qualified readers or interpreters

ADEA

The Age Discrimination in Employment Act of 1967 (ADEA) forbids age discrimination against people who are age 40 or older. It does not protect workers under the age of 40, although some states have laws that protect younger workers from age discrimination. It is not illegal for an employer or other covered entity to favor an older worker over a younger one, even if both workers are age 40 or older. Discrimination can occur when the victim and the person who inflicted the discrimination are both over 40.[6]

The ADEA applies to employers with 20 or more employees. Employers can still discharge any employee regardless of age for legitimate nondiscriminatory reasons. Additionally, the ADEA has an exception that allows employers to discriminate on the basis of age for safety reasons referred to as a bona fide occupational qualification.

EPA

The Equal Pay Act of 1963 prohibits pay discrimination based on gender. It requires employers to provide equal pay for equal work, regardless of gender. Healthcare organizations should conduct regular pay equity audits, address any disparities and promote transparency in pay practices to ensure compliance with the EPA.[7]

The jobs need not be identical, but they must be substantially equal in skill, effort, responsibility and working conditions. The job content, rather than the job title, determines whether jobs are substantially equal.

PDA

The Pregnancy Discrimination Act of 1978 prohibits discrimination based on pregnancy, childbirth, or related medical conditions. It requires employers to treat pregnancy-related conditions the same as other temporary disabilities.[8]

HR must educate leadership in medical practices on age-related biases, implement fair employment practices and address age-related discrimination complaints promptly. One important resource for HR to consider is the Uniform Guidelines on Employee Selection Procedures. Adopted by the EEOC, these guidelines make up a selection process designed to not adversely impact identities protected under the EEOC. The guidelines safeguard against any recruitment tools that may disproportionately screen out such protected individuals from the selection process.

Exhibit 7.1 EEO Case Review

Kaiser Foundation Health Plan of Georgia, Inc., a managed healthcare provider (part of Kaiser Permanente organization) agreed to pay $130,000 to settle an ADA lawsuit in which an employee, whose disabilities made it traumatic for her to access her workplace through revolving doors, had requested to use the available non-revolving doors as a reasonable accommodation. Kaiser refused and forced the employee to use the revolving doors.

Notably, the court held that a reasonable accommodation need not relate to the performance of an essential function of the job; employees with disabilities are also entitled to accommodations to access the workplace and to enjoy the same benefits and privileges of employment as other employees. In addition to monetary relief, Kaiser agreed to train its employees on the ADA, make changes to its employment forms, and allow the EEOC to monitor how it handles future requests for accommodation under the ADA.[9]

7.3 Wage and Hours Laws

FLSA

The Fair Labor Standards Act of 1938 (FLSA) establishes minimum wage, overtime pay, recordkeeping, and youth employment standards affecting employees in the private sector as well as in Federal, State, and local governments. The FLSA covers the following:

Minimum Wage: The federal minimum wage is $7.25 per hour. Many states also have minimum wage laws. In cases where an employee is subject to both state and federal minimum wage laws, the employee is entitled to the higher minimum wage.

Overtime: Covered nonexempt employees must receive overtime pay for hours worked that are over 40 per workweek at a rate not less than one and one-half times the regular rate of pay. There is no limit on the number of hours employees 16 years or older may work in any workweek. The FLSA does not require overtime pay for work on weekends, holidays, or regular days of rest, unless overtime is worked on such days.

Hours Worked: Hours worked ordinarily include all the time during which an employee is required to be on the employer's premises, on duty, or at a prescribed workplace.

Recordkeeping: Employers must display an official poster outlining the requirements of the FLSA. Employers must also keep employee time and pay records.

Child Labor: These provisions are designed to protect the educational opportunities of minors and prohibit their employment in jobs and under conditions detrimental to their health or well-being.[10]

It is important to note that some employees are exempt from the FLSA, meaning they are not eligible for overtime. To be considered "exempt," employees must be paid at least $455 per week and perform the following duties:

- Involving management and/or general business operations of the organization
- Requiring specialized academic training in a computer field
- Selling the organization's services outside the place of business

It is HR's responsibility to stay up to date on labor laws and regulations to ensure that the practice is in compliance. HR teams must also correctly classify workers according to applicable labor laws and should conduct regular audits of timekeeping and payroll practices. By complying with labor laws, such as above, HR teams can minimize the risk of legal disputes and penalties as well as mitigate the risk of misclassification claims.

When conducting an FLSA audit—whether internally or with the help of a third party—consider the following key areas:

- **Employee Classifications:** Review the classification of your employees as exempt or non-exempt under the FLSA guidelines. Ensure that job duties and salaries align with the appropriate classification.
- **Pay Calculations:** Verify that all clinical and administrative staff are receiving at least minimum wage and overtime pay in accordance with federal regulations. Check if there are any miscalculations or inconsistencies in payroll records.
- **Records and Policies:** Examine your recordkeeping practices to confirm that accurate timecards, pay stubs and other necessary documents are being maintained. Assess whether policies regarding breaks, meal periods and time off comply with FLSA requirements.
- **Independent Contractors:** Evaluate any independent contractors working for your business to determine if they meet the criteria set by the FLSA for proper classification.
- **Compliance Training:** Make sure managers and HR personnel receive regular training on FLSA regulations to stay updated on any changes in labor laws.[11]

Exhibit 7.2 FLSA Case Review

The U.S. Department of Labor obtained a federal court order requiring an Illinois home healthcare provider to pay 69 workers $1.1 million in back wages and damages for its failure to pay these workers for all hours worked. U.S. District Court Judge Colin Bruce for the Central District of Illinois in Urbana issued an order finding the owner and operator liable for back wages and damages.

The court's action follows an investigation by the department's Wage and Hour Division that the practice paid a daily rate to workers employed as caregivers, the majority of whom worked 24-hour shifts, regardless of the number of hours they worked, resulting in minimum wage and overtime violations. The caregivers provided in-home healthcare and assisted living services to clients across Mattoon, Champaign and Tuscola. The investigation determined that the employer owed the affected workers $562,389 in back wages and assessed an equal amount of liquidated damages.

The court also ruled the practice violated the FLSA's recordkeeping requirements by failing to track an employee's hours worked, including sleep time interruptions, accurately. By failing to do so, the organization's sleep credit was invalid. Following the department's investigation, the practice changed their payroll practices effective Jan. 4, 2021, and began paying workers on an hourly basis and computing overtime for hours over 40 in a workweek.[12]

7.4 Employee Benefits Laws

HIPAA

The Health Insurance Portability and Accountability Act of 1996 HIPAA) is a federal law that requires the creation of national standards to protect sensitive patient health information from being disclosed without the patient's consent or knowledge. The US Department of Health and Human Services (HHS) issued the HIPAA Privacy Rule to implement the requirements of HIPAA.[13]

HIPAA Privacy Rule

The Privacy Rule standards address the use and disclosure of individuals' health information known as protected health information (PHI) by entities subject to the Privacy Rule. These individuals and organizations are called "covered entities."

The Privacy Rule also contains standards for individuals' rights to understand and control how their health information is used. A major goal of the Privacy Rule is to make sure that individuals' health information is properly protected while allowing the flow of health information needed to provide and promote high-quality healthcare, and to protect the public's health and well-being. The Privacy Rule permits important uses of information while protecting the privacy of people who seek care and healing.

HIPAA Security Rule

While the HIPAA Privacy Rule safeguards protected health information (PHI), the Security Rule protects a subset of information covered by the Privacy Rule. This subset is all individually identifiable health information a covered entity creates, receives, maintains or transmits in electronic form. This information is called electronic protected health information (e-PHI). The Security Rule does not apply to PHI transmitted orally or in writing.

FMLA

The Family and Medical Leave Act of 1993 provides job-protected, unpaid leave for medical and family reasons. It allows eligible employees to take up to 12 weeks of leave without employment consequences. Eligibility is determined by being employed with the employer for at least a year and working at least 1,250 hours over the past 12 months.[14]

FMLA requires employers with 50 or more employees to provide up to 12 weeks for employees to take care of a new child, take care of a seriously ill immediate family member (parent, spouse or child), or to take care of one's own serious health condition.

Many states have enacted laws with additional mandates to FMLA. These additional mandates include compliance for organizations with fewer employees along with an expanded definition of immediate family that includes domestic partners and their children, grandparents and in-laws. It's important that your medical practice complies with your state's up-to-date FMLA mandates.

ACA

The Affordable Care Act of 2010 (ACA) was enacted to expand the availability and coverage of affordable health insurance. The law provides consumers with subsidies ("premium tax credits") that lower costs for households with incomes between 100% - 400% of the federal poverty line (FPL). ACA also expands the Medicaid program to cover all adults with income below 138% of the FPL. It's also designed to support the innovation of medical care delivery methods that may help lower health-care costs.[15]

If you have fewer than 25 full-time employees, including full-time equivalent employees, you may be eligible for a Small Business Health Care Tax Credit to help cover the cost of providing coverage.

If you have 50 or more full-time employees, including full-time equivalent employees, you are an applicable full-time employer and need to issue statements to employees and file an annual information return reporting whether and what health insurance you offered employees. Healthcare organizations should track employee hours, conduct affordability tests, and stay updated on IRS reporting forms and deadlines. It is also important to communicate with employees about their rights and responsibilities.

Complying with the ACA can be a challenge for small practices, as there are frequent rule changes along with many details to consider. Ensure compliance by working with an experienced insurance broker who can help you navigate the law and find the best health insurance coverage for your practice.

The ACA affects the use of Health Savings Accounts (HSA) and Flexible Spending Account (FSA). HSAs are typically owned by the employee who is enrolled in a high-deductible health plan. As the employee makes contributions up to the tax deadline for that year, the HSA has investment capability. FSAs, on the other hand, are owned by the employer who must offer a group health plan. The employee can choose their contribution amount at the start of the year, but FSAs have no potential for investment by the employee.

Exhibit 7.3 Health Savings Account vs Flexible Spending Account

HSA Health Savings Account	VS	FSA Flexible Spending Account
Owned by the employee		Owned by the employer
Must be enrolled in a high-deductible health plan		Must be offered a group health plan by the employer
Contributions can be made until tax day for the year		Choose your contribution amount at the start of the year
Investment capability		No investment capability

Consider the following to ensure compliance with the ACA:

- **Determine if you're required to be compliant:** You may be exempt from the employer shared responsibility provision if you have 50 or fewer full-time equivalent employees.
- **Have an appropriate waiting period:** All group health plans must have a waiting period that does not exceed 90 days and an orientation period that does not exceed one month.
- **Watch what you put a dollar limit on:** No annual dollar limits can be placed on coverage of "essential health benefits" (EHBs).
- **Check maximum out-of-pocket costs:** EHBs provided by group health plans in-network have limits on annual out-of-pocket costs for individuals ($9,100) and family coverage ($18,200).
- **Check your health reimbursement arrangements:** Small practices with a Health Reimbursement Arrangement (HRA) must comply with rules including a limit on money put into the account and types of expenses that can be reimbursed.
- **Analyze your Health Flexible Spending Arrangements (FSAs):** No participant can receive benefits exceeding double their annual salary reduction election, or $500 plus their salary reduction if that is greater.
- **Determine if you'll allow carryover of FSA money:** Decide if you want to allow employees to carry over leftover

health FSA money into the next plan year then make the appropriate changes to your company's healthcare policy.

- **Understand HSA payment opportunities.** You can use HSA funds to pay for deductibles, copayments, coinsurance and other qualified medical expenses.
- **Know the HSA rollover.** Unspent HSA funds roll over from year to year, allowing you to build tax-free savings to pay for medical care later.
- **Send notices to employees within 14 days of hire:** This written notice must include details about the Health Insurance Marketplace and provide a Summary of Benefits and Coverage along with Notice of Plan Changes.
- **Offer minimum essential coverage:** All group health plans must provide minimum essential coverage, which is a defined set of benefits that must be met in order for a plan to be ACA compliant.
- **Have an affordable coverage option:** All group health plans must offer at least one health insurance option with a premium that doesn't exceed 9.12% of an employee's household income.
- **Use forms 1094 and 1095 to report coverage:** Applicable Large Employers must use forms 1094 and 1095 to report health coverage information to the IRS.[16]

COBRA

The Consolidated Omnibus Budget Reconciliation Act of 1985 (COBRA) gives workers and their families who lose their health benefits the right to choose to continue group health benefits provided by their group health plan for limited periods of time under certain circumstances such as voluntary or involuntary job loss, reduction in hours worked, transition between jobs, death, divorce and other life events. Qualified individuals may be required to pay the entire premium for coverage up to 102% of the cost to the plan.[17]

COBRA generally requires that group health plans sponsored by employers with 20 or more employees in the prior year offer employees and their families the opportunity for a temporary extension of health coverage (called continuation coverage) in certain instances where coverage under the plan would otherwise end.

COBRA outlines how employees and family members may elect continuation coverage. It also requires employers and plans to provide notice. It is up to the HR department to provide timely and accurate information to employees about their rights under COBRA, and ensure compliance with notification and administrative requirements.

ERISA

The Employee Retirement Income Security Act of 1974 (ERISA) is a federal law that sets minimum standards for most voluntarily established retirement and health plans in private industry to provide protection for individuals in these plans.[18]

ERISA requires plans to provide participants with plan information including important information about plan features and funding; sets minimum standards for participation, vesting, benefit accrual and funding; provides fiduciary responsibilities for those who manage and control plan assets; requires plans to establish a grievance and appeals process for participants to get benefits from their plans; gives participants the right to sue for benefits and breaches of fiduciary duty; and, if a defined benefits plan is terminated, guarantees payment of certain benefits through a federally chartered corporation, known as the Pension Benefit Guaranty Corporation (PBGC).

In general, ERISA does not cover plans established or maintained by governmental entities or plans which are maintained solely to comply with applicable workers compensation, unemployment or disability laws. ERISA also does not cover plans maintained outside the United States primarily for the benefit of nonresident aliens or unfunded excess benefits plans.

Some states allow employers with up to 100 employees to buy coverage through the Small Business Health Options Program, or SHOP Marketplace. Regardless of size, all employers that provide self-insured health coverage to employees must file an annual return reporting certain information for each covered employee and provide the same information to covered individuals.

In order for healthcare organizations to ensure compliance to ERISA regulations, HR leadership must communicate benefits to staff and conduct regular audits of benefits plans.

Exhibit 7.3 HIPAA Case Review

A private multi-specialty physician group with approximately 150 locations in New Jersey and Southern Connecticut. In the Fall of 2021, the Office for Civil Rights (OCR) received six complaints from individuals who had not been provided with their records after sending a request to the group. The requests were to obtain a copy of an individual's own records or requests from parents for copies of their minor children's records.

The HIPAA Privacy Rule gives individuals the right to obtain a copy of their medical records and those of their minor children. When a request is received by a HIPAA covered entity, the records must be provided within 30 calendar days, although under certain limited circumstances, a 30-day extension is possible. OCR launched an investigation in response to the complaints and determined that the practice had exceeded the allowed timeframe for providing those records. The complainants had to wait between 84 days and 231 days to receive their requested records.

The physician group chose to settle the alleged violations and agreed to pay a $160,000 financial penalty and adopt a corrective action plan (CAP) that includes reviewing and revising its policies and procedures for individual access to PHI, providing training to the workforce on those new procedures, and ensuring that all patients are provided with their requested records within 30 days.[19]

7.5 Immigration Laws

INA

The body of law governing U.S. immigration policy is called the Immigration and Nationality Act of 1952 (INA). The INA allows the United States to grant up to 675,000 permanent immigrant visas each year across various visa categories. On top of those 675,000 visas, the INA sets no limit on the annual admission of U.S. citizens' spouses, parents and children under the age of 21. In addition, each year the president is required to consult with Congress and set an annual number of refugees to be admitted to the United States through the U.S. Refugee Admissions Program.[20]

Once a person obtains an immigrant visa and comes to the United States, they become a lawful permanent resident (LPR). In some circumstances, noncitizens already inside the United States can obtain LPR status through a process known as "adjustment of status."

LPRs are eligible to apply for nearly all jobs and can remain in the country permanently, even if they are unemployed. After residing in the United States for five years (or three years in some circumstances), LPRs are eligible to apply for U.S. citizenship. It is impossible to apply for citizenship through the normal process without first becoming an LPR.

IRCA

The Immigration Reform and Control Act of 1986 prohibits employers from hiring unauthorized workers and requires employers to verify identity and employment eligibility of their employees.[21]

I-9 Verification

Use Form I-9 to verify the identity and employment authorization of individuals hired for employment in the United States. All U.S. employers must properly complete Form I-9 for every individual they hire for employment in the United States. This includes citizens and noncitizens. Both employees and employers (or authorized representatives of the employer) must complete the form.[22]

On the form, an employee must attest to their employment authorization. The employee must also present their employer with acceptable documents as evidence of identity and employment authorization. The employer must examine these documents to determine whether they reasonably appear to be genuine and relate to the employee, then record the document information on the employee's Form I-9. Certain employers who choose to remotely examine the employee's documentation under a DHS-authorized alternative procedure rather than via physical examination must indicate they did so by checking the box provided.

HR is responsible for ensuring proper documentation for employment eligibility, conducting I-9 audits and staying informed about immigration compliance issues.

7.6 Workforce Safety Laws

OSHA

With the Occupational Safety and Health Act of 1970, Congress created the Occupational Safety and Health Administration (OSHA) to ensure safe and healthful working conditions for workers by setting and enforcing standards as well as providing training, outreach, education and assistance.[23]

Employers have the responsibility to provide a safe workplace. Employers must provide their workers with a workplace that does not have serious hazards and must follow all OSHA safety and health standards. Employers must find and correct safety and health problems. OSHA further requires that employers must first try to eliminate or reduce hazards by making reasonable changes in working conditions rather than relying on personal protective equipment such as masks, gloves or earplugs.

Through HR, medical practices can ensure compliance with OSHA standards and maintain a safe and compliant work environment with these methods:

- Creating and implementing written safety plans
- Providing personal protective equipment (PPE) when necessary
- Develop safety committees with staff
- Conduct regular safety training

Both clinical and administrative staff will be more aware and engaged in their workplace environment when they are included in the process of ensuring safety and compliance.

Exhibit 7.4 OSHA Case Review

A provider of inpatient and outpatient behavioral healthcare based in Middleton, Wis., was fined $8,370 by OSHA following an investigation of an incident where a nurse was accidentally spiked with a needle stick to establish whether the healthcare provider was compliant with safety and health regulations.

The incident occurred in December 2022 and did not result in any loss of work time or patient safety impacts; however, OSHA's inspection identified safety and health failures resulting in four citations, three of which were serious and related to safety and health risks. The citations included a failure to maintain a proper work injury log, a failure to properly record the needle stick incident in its injury log, and a failure to include certain jobs in its exposure control plan.

All of the citations were fully abated within 24 hours and were mostly related to documentation issues. A spokesperson for the provider confirmed that its documentation policy has now been updated and further training has been provided to employees to ensure full compliance in the future. The citations were resolved through an informal settlement with OSHA in June 2023.[24]

7.7 Other Laws

NLRA

In 1935, Congress passed the National Labor Relations Act ("NLRA"). The NLRA governs relations between employers, employees and labor unions. It protects the employee's right to organize, join unions, strike and collectively bargain. Healthcare organizations should train supervisors on NLRA rights and prohibited practices and ensure consistent application of policies during union activity.[25]

By staying informed about employee's rights and addressing labor relations issues promptly, HR leadership can ensure fair labor practices in the workplace.

Wrongful Discharge/Termination Laws

Wrongful discharge refers to the unlawful termination of an employee, and it can include issues such as discrimination, retaliation, or violation of employment contracts. Most states are at-will states, except Montana, which means that an employer or employee can terminate their employment for any reason, with or without notice, as long as it isn't a violation to labor laws. To strategically address these concerns, HR professionals should proactively establish clear and consistent termination policies, ensuring alignment with federal, state and local employment laws.[26]

Developing transparent communication channels and documentation procedures is crucial to support the organization's decisions and provide a defense against potential legal claims. HR should conduct regular training sessions for managers on proper termination procedures, emphasizing the importance of fairness, consistency and adherence to established policies. Moreover, staying informed about changes in employment laws, consulting legal counsel when necessary and implementing ethical practices throughout the employment lifecycle are key components of a strategic approach to wrongful discharge prevention and compliance. This proactive stance not only safeguards the organization from legal risks but also fosters a positive workplace culture built on fairness and accountability.

Below are some measures that can reduce the risk of liability regarding termination:

- Develop a written policy that clearly covers the grounds for termination.
- Include specific disclaimers in job application forms, policy materials and employee handbooks explaining that these documents are not an employee contract.
- Educate managers about the importance of logging and documenting every termination action.
- Ensure that your practice's performance review forms and job descriptions accurately reflect expectations (performance, objectives, behaviors, goals).

- Reinforce to managers the importance of warning employees in advance when actions can lead to possible termination.
- Train managers to stay alert for signs of poor performance.
- Communicate to managers frequently that termination of an employee is not solely their decision.
- Consider offering a severance package that includes limited continuation of benefits.
- Consider purchasing defense and judgment insurance to protect employees against lawsuits.
- Conduct training for managers and supervisors on both their responsibilities and employee rights.
- Terminate employees only as a last resort with great care and compassion.

7.8 State Law vs. Federal Law

It is important for an organization's HR department to stay up to date on both state and federal laws. Federal laws are created and administered nationally for all states and typically set the minimum of what is required, however state laws may have additional requirements or modifications that fit the specific needs of the state. When state and federal laws conflict, Federal law preempts state law, according to the Supremacy Clause of the U.S. Constitution. Keep this in mind when establishing policies and procedures for your organization.

7.9 Summary

Medical practices should proactively stay informed about changes in legislation, conduct regular training for employees and managers, implement policies and procedures that align with legal requirements, and respond promptly to employee concerns or complaints. Having documentation on clear and concise policies and procedures is vital to communicating laws and regulations throughout your organization. Whether it be an employee handbook, a policies manual or an internal intranet, having such resources will help you and your staff's ability to comply with current and long standing employment laws and regulations.

To summarize, here are some key strategies for a healthcare organizations' HR departments to follow that can reduce risk and ensure compliance:

- Review employee handbooks, job descriptions, I-9 forms, and other HR documentation to ensure they align with current labor laws and regulations.
- Ensure that the handbook clearly outlines employee rights, expectations and procedures, reducing the risk of misunderstandings or legal disputes.
- Conduct regular workshops, webinars, or training sessions to educate stakeholders about their rights and responsibilities, preventing unintentional violations.
- Ensure accurate and detailed records related to employee performance, disciplinary actions, accommodation requests, and other HR processes.
- Conduct regular training sessions on diversity, equity, and inclusion, and promptly investigate and address any complaints to prevent legal claims.
- Regularly communicate changes in HR policies, legal updates, and organizational initiatives to ensure employees are well-informed and can voice concerns early.
- Conduct periodic audits of employee classifications (exempt vs. non-exempt), track hours worked accurately and ensure proper payment of overtime when applicable.
- Clearly communicate whistleblower protections, provide channels for anonymous reporting, and investigate complaints promptly and thoroughly.
- Train HR staff and managers on conflict resolution techniques, encourage open communication, and provide mediation services when necessary.
- Develop a relationship with legal counsel to obtain guidance on complex HR issues, ensuring that decisions align with legal requirements.
- Establish clear procedures for employees to request accommodations, engage in an interactive process and document the efforts made to provide reasonable accommodations.

The next and final chapter will discuss key KPIs and scenarios in which healthcare organizations can leverage such KPIs into their HR strategy.

Resources

- **eLawsAdvisor:** www.dol.gov/elaws/advisors.html
- **Wage and Hour Division Website:** www.dol.gov/mhd
- **Equal Employment Opportunity Commission Website:** www.eeoc.gov
- **Uniform Guidelines on Employee Selection Procedures:** https://www.uniformguidelines.com/

Notes

1. HR Digest. https://www.thehrdigest.com/hr-compliance-staying-compliant-with-changing-labor-laws-and-regulations/
2. DOL. https://www.dol.gov/general/topic/discrimination
3. EEOC. https://www.eeoc.gov/overview
4. FTC. https://www.ftc.gov/policy-notices/no-fear-act/protections-against-discrimination
5. EEOC. https://www.eeoc.gov/publications/ada-your-responsibilities-employer
6. EEOC. https://www.eeoc.gov/age-discrimination
7. EEOC. https://www.eeoc.gov/statutes/equal-pay-act-1963
8. EEOC. https://www.eeoc.gov/statutes/pregnancy-discrimination-act-1978
9. EEOC. https://www.eeoc.gov/select-list-resolved-cases-involving-mental-health-conditions-under-ada-may-2022
10. DOL. https://www.dol.gov/agencies/whd/flsa
11. Onsi Group. https://www.onsigroup.com/blog/what-is-an-flsa-audit
12. DOL. https://www.dol.gov/newsroom/releases/whd/whd20230221-1
13. CDC. https://www.cdc.gov/phlp/publications/topic/hipaa.html
14. DOL. https://www.dol.gov/general/topic/benefits-leave/fmla
15. IRS. https://www.irs.gov/affordable-care-act/employers
16. Forbes. https://www.forbes.com/advisor/business/aca-compliance/
17. DOL. https://www.dol.gov/general/topic/health-plans/cobra
18. DOL. https://www.dol.gov/general/topic/retirement/erisa
19. HIPAA Journal. https://www.hipaajournal.com/optum-medical-care-new-jersey-hipaa-settlement/

20. American Immigration Council. https://www.americanimmigrationcouncil.org/research/how-united-states-immigration-system-works
21. Congress.gov https://www.congress.gov/bill/99th-congress/senate-bill/1200/text
22. USCIS. https://www.uscis.gov/i-9
23. OSHA. https://www.osha.gov/aboutosha
24. HIPAA Journal. https://www.hipaajournal.com/osha-issues-citations-to-florida-and-wisconsin-hospitals-for-health-and-safety-failures/
25. National Labor Relations Board. https://www.nlrb.gov/guidance/key-reference-materials/national-labor-relations-act
26. USA.gov https://www.usa.gov/wrongful-termination

Chapter 8

Leveraging KPIs in HR Strategic Processes

8.1 Combining KPIs with Strategic Thinking

In today's dynamic healthcare landscape, HR plays a pivotal role in shaping the success of healthcare systems. HR strategic processes are no longer confined to administrative tasks; they are integral to driving organizational growth, employee engagement and patient outcomes. One of the cornerstones of effective HR strategic planning is the use of Key Performance Indicators (KPIs), which provide actionable insights and data-driven decision-making. This chapter explores how practices can harness the power of KPIs to enhance their HR strategic processes and foster a culture of continuous improvement.

Role of KPIs in HR Strategic Thinking

As discussed earlier, HR strategic thinking involves aligning HR practices with broader organizational goals to create a thriving workplace culture and drive organizational performance. It requires a proactive approach to anticipate future talent needs, address workforce challenges and position the organization as a preferred employer. Strategic thinking in HR goes beyond reacting to immediate needs; it involves long-term planning to ensure sustainable success.

Effective HR strategic planning in a healthcare system involves monitoring and measuring various key performance indicators (KPIs) that reflect the organization's workforce, talent management and overall HR-related goals. By comparing in-house numbers with industry standards, organizations can spot opportunities for growth and create a retention strategy.

KPIs are quantifiable metrics that help measure performance and progress toward organizational objectives. They provide a clear and objective way to assess the effectiveness of HR initiatives, make informed decisions and course correct as needed. When applied to HR strategic thinking, KPIs offer a comprehensive view of the workforce, allowing HR professionals to identify strengths, areas for improvement and strategic opportunities.

In a 2009 paper *Performance Management Strategies*, Wayne W. Eckerson describes a number of characteristics of "good" KPIs and mentions that a KPI should be related to a desired business outcome and that KPIs "shouldn't undermine each other."[1] According to Eckerson, effective KPIs include the following characteristics:

- **Sparse:** The fewer KPIs, the better
- **Drillable:** Users can drill into detail
- **Simple:** Users understand the KPIs
- **Actionable:** Users know how to affect outcomes
- **Owned:** KPIs have an owner
- **Referenced:** Users can view origins and context
- **Correlated:** KPIs drive desired outcomes
- **Balanced:** KPIs consist of both financial and non-financial metrics
- **Aligned:** KPIs don't undermine each other
- **Validated:** Workers can't circumvent the KPIs

Too often, leaders get caught up in identifying too many key performance indicators (KPIs) and managing data that needs to be more relevant.

The key to successful business analytics is to ensure the KPIs are tied to the desired outcomes. Another way to think about it is to identify the behavior that needs to be changed and make that factor the KPI for measurement. Now, what processes need to be in place to obtain that information? Overall, the idea is to identify, collect and use pertinent information to benchmark positive or negative performance related to achieving desired outcomes.

Ultimately ask, "How can HR prove that its involvement in organizational goals will produce positive results?" With metrics, a practice can prove the effect a position and department has on the organization's people and, thus, its performance. To get started with business intelligence and business analytics, identify the organization's current state of affairs and the existing measurements, then identify an area on which to concentrate.

8.2 Key Steps in Integrating KPIs into HR Strategic Processes

Leveraging HR KPIs for strategic growth in a medical practice involves a systematic approach to measure, analyze and improve HR-related processes that affect the organization's overall success. KPIs allow a medical practice to make data-driven decisions and thus strategically position itself for sustainable growth in a competitive healthcare environment. Below are key steps for integrating KPIs into HR's strategic process.

1. **Define organization objectives**
   - Align HR goals with overarching objectives of the healthcare system or the medical practice's strategic objectives.
   - Identify specific HR outcomes that directly affect the achievement of these objectives.

2. **Selective relevant KPIs**
   - Choose KPIs that reflect critical aspects of HR, i.e. employee engagement, turnover rates, talent acquisition, training effectiveness, patient satisfaction, etc.
   - KPIs should be measurable, relevant and directly tied to strategic goals.

3. Data collection and analytics

- Gather accurate and timely data related to the selected KPIs.
- Regularly analyze the data to identify trends, patterns and areas requiring attention.
- Use automated HR systems to streamline data gathering and minimize errors.

4. Benchmarking and comparison

- Compare KPIs against industry benchmarks and best practices to assess the organization's performance.
- Benchmarking provides insights into areas where the organization excels and areas where improvements are needed.

5. Setting targets and goals

- Establish realistic targets and goals for each KPI based on the organization's strategic priorities using historical data, industry benchmarks, and growth projections.
- Clear targets provide a framework for tracking progress and performance improvement.

6. Action planning

- Develop action plans to address areas of concern identified through KPI analysis.
- Focus on strategies that drive positive change and contribute to the organization's strategic success.

7. Continuous monitoring and reporting

- Regularly monitor KPIs to track progress toward goals.
- Analyze trends, identify patterns and pinpoint areas that need attention.
- Provide stakeholders, including leadership, managers and employees with transparent and data-driven reports to facilitate decision-making.
- Be prepared to adjust strategies based on new data and changing circumstances.

KPIs provide insights into areas such as workforce stability, talent development, employee well-being, diversity and inclusion efforts, compliance and recruitment effectiveness. By tracking these metrics, healthcare systems can make informed decisions, set strategic priorities and continually enhance their HR strategies to align with organizational goals.

8.3 Essential KPIs for healthcare systems' HR strategic plans

Consider the following KPIs that are essential to integrating into any health system's or medical practices HR strategy.[2]

Exhibit 8.1 KPIs for HR Strategy

KPIs	Description	Measurement/ Calculation	Strategy
Compliance and Training Effectiveness	Ensuring that an organization maintains legal and ethical standards, minimizing risks, and promoting a culture of continuous learning and development.	Measuring improvements in performance after training and well as completion rates.	Provides data and insights that enable HR and leadership teams to make informed decisions about program improvements, content updates, and resource allocation.
Absenteeism Rate	Percentage of scheduled work hours that employees miss due to absences.	Number of absences/number of work days	Allows an organization to proactively address issues related to employee engagement, well-being and workforce planning.
Employee engagement	Measurement of employees' emotional commitment to their work and the organization.	Employee Satisfaction Surveys to gather feedback on various aspects of the workplace experience.	Monitoring employee engagement is crucial as it affects workplace productivity, talent retention, patient satisfaction and innovation. Engaged employees are more likely to contribute positively to the organization's mission and achieve strategic objectives.

KPIs	Description	Measurement/ Calculation	Strategy
Health and Wellness Metrics	Should align with the organization's overall goals and strategies for promoting a healthier and more productive workforce	Absenteeism, employee satisfaction and participation in wellness program	Allows organizations to make informed decisions, refine wellness programs, and prioritize initiatives that have the greatest influence on employee health and well-being
Employee Turnover Rate	Percentage of employees who leave the organization over a specific time period	Turnover rate(%)=(number of leavers/Avg. number of employees)x100	Provides insights into employee satisfaction, organizational culture and retention efforts
Retention of Talent	The ability an organization has to keep its employees	(Remaining headcount during set period/headcount at the start of the period) x100	Positions organizations for long-term planning and strategic growth by focusing on innovation and expansion
Average Tenure	Average length of time employees remain with the organization	Total employment time for all employees/ Total number of employees hired	Reflects job satisfaction and organizational commitment
Promotion and Internal Mobility	Percentage of promotions filled internally	Total number of internal movements/ total number of employees x100	Reflects opportunities for career advancement within the organization
Vacancy Rate	Percentage of open positions compared to the total number of authorized positions	(Number of vacant positions/ Total number of positions) x100	Indicates staffing gaps that need to be addressed while allowing for trend analysis

KPIs	Description	Measurement/ Calculation	Strategy
Talent Acquisition Metrics	Evaluating the effectiveness of different recruitment sources as well as calculating the percentage of candidates who move from one recruitment stage to the next	Number of candidates generated from the channel during a given timeframe and compare which channel is producing the most (quantity/quality) candidates(Sourcing Channel Effectiveness Calculation)	Helps an organization attract and retain the best talent, allocation resources to the most productive channels, thus optimizing recruitment strategies. **Conversion Rate Calculation:** Number of candidates from the pipeline that were interviewed/ number of candidates that were recommended to the recruiter/manage
Cost per Hire	Total cost associated with recruiting and hiring a new employee	(External cost + Internal cost)/ Total number of hires	Provides insights into recruitment efficiency and cost-effectiveness
Training and Development Investments	Percentage of the HR budget allocated to employee training and development	Amount of dollars used for training and development vs what was budgeted	Reflects commitment to skill enhancement and career growth

8.4 Benefits of KPI-Driven HR Strategic Thinking

KPI-driven strategic thinking in healthcare HR brings forth a range of significant advantages. By harnessing KPIs, HR professionals gain real-time insights that facilitate informed decision-making, allowing them to promptly address emerging challenges and implement necessary improvements. This proactive approach enables healthcare organizations to stay ahead of trends, regulatory changes, and workforce demands, ensuring operational efficiency and agility in a dynamic healthcare landscape.[3]

Aligning HR initiatives with organizational goals and KPIs tied to these objectives guide the strategic direction. By establishing clear and measurable KPIs that reflect key organizational priorities, HR professionals can effectively communicate the value of HR initiatives to senior leadership and stakeholders. This alignment fosters a culture of accountability and performance-driven decision-making, enhancing the organization's ability to achieve its strategic objectives and drive sustainable growth.[4]

KPI-driven HR strategic thinking enables healthcare organizations to optimize resource allocation and maximize return on investment (ROI) in HR initiatives. By identifying KPIs related to workforce productivity, engagement and retention, HR professionals can allocate resources strategically to areas that have the greatest effect on organizational performance. This data-driven approach empowers healthcare organizations to optimize staffing levels, invest in employee development programs, and implement targeted recruitment strategies to attract and retain top talent.[5]

8.5 Practice in Action

Below are scenarios using KPIs and the role in which HR works with healthcare leaders to further the organization's strategic goals. These scenarios showcase how medical practice leadership can utilize HR KPIs as critical decision-making tools to guide strategic direction, optimize operations, enhance patient care, control costs and ensure long-term success in the healthcare industry. The proactive identification of potential issues through KPIs empowers HR to take preemptive measures, thereby promoting stability and preventing escalations. The benefits extend to the workforce, fostering an enriched employee experience.

Exhibit 8.2 Healthcare Scenarios for HR KPIs

KPIs	Scenario	Measurement/ Calculation	Strategy
Workforce Planning	The organization is expanding its primary care services to meet the needs of an aging population	Population demographics, projected patient volumes, physician-to-patient ratios	HR collaborates with operations to determine the number of primary care providers needed, along with recruitment strategies and timelines

KPIs	Scenario	Measurement/ Calculation	Strategy
Employee and Provider Engagement and Retention	Employee engagement scores have decreased significantly in the last quarter	Employee engagement survey results, turnover rate, employee satisfaction scores	HR decides to implement initiatives to improve engagement, such as leadership training, flexible work arrangements, or wellness programs
Compensation and Benefits	The organization wants to attract top-tier talent in a highly competitive market	Compensation surveys, turnover rates, benefits utilization	HR recommends revising the compensation structure and expanding benefits packages to remain competitive
Talent Acquisition and Recruitment	The healthcare organization is experiencing a high turnover rate among nurses	Turnover rate, time-to-fill vacancies, cost-per-hire	HR identifies the need to invest in recruitment strategies to reduce turnover, such as improving the onboarding process and offering competitive compensation packages
Succession Planning	Several key leaders in the organization are nearing retirement	Leadership assessments, retirement projections, internal talent pipeline	HR works on identifying and developing potential successors, creating a seamless transition plan for leadership positions
Training and Development	The organization faces a skills gap in its IT department	Skills assessment scores, training completion rates, skill acquisition speed	HR recommends investing in targeted training programs to upskill the IT team, ensuring they have the necessary skills for the organization's digital transformation
Compliance and Risk Management	The organization faces potential legal challenges related to HR practices	Compliance audit results, employee relations data, litigation history	*Collaboration:* HR advises on implementing policies and procedures that mitigate legal risks and ensure compliance with labor laws and regulations

8.6 Summary

It is important to remember that each medical practice and healthcare organization is unique and different, necessitating careful attention to determining appropriate data to utilize when performing benchmarking analysis. In the healthcare industry, where patient care and outcomes are paramount, effective HR strategic thinking supported by KPIs is essential for building a strong, engaged workforce. By integrating KPIs into HR strategic processes, healthcare systems can foster a culture of continuous improvement, adapt to changing industry trends and position themselves for sustainable success in a dynamic healthcare landscape. KPIs provide the analytical foundation upon which HR can guide the organization toward its goals while delivering optimal care to patients and cultivating a fulfilling work environment for employees.

Key points discussed in this chapter include:

- Effective HR strategic planning in a healthcare system involves monitoring and measuring various (KPIs) that reflect the organization's workforce, talent management and overall HR-related goals.
- KPIs allow a medical practice to make data-driven decisions and thus strategically position itself for sustainable growth in a competitive healthcare environment.
- KPIs provide insights into areas such as workforce stability, talent development, employee well-being, diversity and inclusion efforts, compliance and recruitment effectiveness.
- HR can establish itself as a strategic partner in the healthcare organization's success, contributing to high-quality patient care, a motivated workforce and sustainable growth in the dynamic healthcare industry.

KPI-driven HR strategic thinking fosters a culture of continuous improvement and innovation within healthcare organizations. By regularly monitoring and evaluating KPIs, HR professionals can identify areas for improvement, experiment with new approaches and measure the effectiveness of HR interventions over time. HR professionals gain real-time insights that facilitate informed decision-making, allowing them to promptly address these emerging challenges and adapt to changing market conditions, industry trends, and patient needs.

Notes

1. Wayne W. Eckerson https://www.spendit.de/wp-content/uploads/2021/10/TDWI _Performance-Management-Strategies.pdf

2. https://business.linkedin.com/content/dam/me/business/en-us/talent-solutions /resources/ pdfs/cheatsheet-recruiting-metrics-for-smbs_v2.pdf

3. https://www.gartner.com/en/newsroom/04-28-2022-gartner-says-us-total-annual -employee-turnover-will-likely-jump-by-nearly-twenty-percent-from-the-prepandemic -annual-average

4. https://www.mgma.com/datadive/management-and-staff

5. https://www.ncbi.nlm.nih.gov/pmc/articles/PMC9926442/

Conclusion

Volume 2 of MGMA's *Advanced Strategy for Medical Practices* series serves as a comprehensive guide for HR professionals and medical practice leaders to apply strategic planning principles and best practices designed to align with an organization's mission, vision and values. By navigating the landscape of strategic HR management within the healthcare work environment, each chapter has provided insights and actionable strategies to elevate HR functions in a way that fosters organizational excellence while addressing the many challenges faced within the modern healthcare industry.

Through strategic planning, practices can conduct a thorough analysis of business needs and organizational goals to develop a comprehensive HR strategy. Modern challenges to medical staffing require HR professionals to be adept, interactive and inventive in their strategies to help attract, retain and enhance the lives of their employees. For example, embracing a strategic approach to the employment lifecycle—from defining the employee value proposition to conducting comprehensive job analyses—can ensure alignment with business objectives and maximize employee value.

This book also explored ways to enhance an organization's culture through initiatives such as employee recognition, employee engagement and diversity. By emphasizing organizational culture and open communication, practices can promote a safe and inclusive work environment through optimized communication channels. Fostering a culture of continuous improvement can also help practices drive engagement, improve retention and enhance organizational growth. Performance management systems that encourage employee feedback and autonomy can sustainably invest in employee development.

In addition to enhanced employee engagement and development initiatives, designing competitive compensation and benefits programs that are equitable for all organizational levels can help medical groups attract and retain top talent. Performance-based incentives coupled with comprehensive benefits packages can maximize retention in an industry hit hard by turnover. Even the pre-employment phase up to a new hire's first 90 days can provide important opportunities for healthcare organizations to apply strategic HR practices. Streamlining the hiring process, conducting engaging interviews and providing comprehensive onboarding programs can help facilitate seamless transitions for new hires, setting up any organization for potential long-term success.

As medical groups continue to embrace modern solutions and technology, data can play a crucial role in strategic HR management. Integrating key performance indicators into the strategic planning processes can help practices leverage data-driven insights to optimize HR functions and drive organizational success. KPIs such as employee turnover rate, time-to-fill vacancies and training effectiveness metrics can measure the success of HR initiatives and inform strategic decision-making.

As organizations implement their HR strategies, staying current on labor laws and regulations are vital to ensuring a compliant and safe workplace while mitigating legal risks. Through clear communication with leadership and staff, along with regular audits of policies and procedures, HR professionals can be proactive in promoting anti-discrimination and harassment initiatives, maintaining accurate and lawful records, and implementing fair wages and work hours.

By embracing these key takeaways and implementing the strategies outlined in this book, forward-thinking HR professionals and medical practice leaders can navigate the complexities and challenges of the healthcare industry with confidence, positioning their organizations for sustained success in a dynamic and competitive landscape. As best practices can vary from one organization to another, these strategies and tools serve as a starting point for establishing your organization's policies and procedures.

Index

comfortable communication, 100
interviewee's career goals, 100
key practices, 99
manage direction & flow, 100
preparation, 100
presentation, 100
Involuntary Separation, 131
IRCA. *See* Immigration Reform and
Control Act of 1986

J
Job Analysis, 45, 60, 68
three elements of, 61

K
Key Performance Indicator, 161
Knowledge, Skills & Attributes, 64
KPI. *See* Key Performance Indicator
healthcare KPI scenarios, 168
KPI Effective Traits, 162
KSA. *See* Knowledge, Skills & Attributes

L
Labor Laws, 139
Lawful Permanent Resident, 153
Leadership Development Disconnect,
117
Leave
Family and Medical Leave Act of
1993, 90, 147
paid time off, 54, 88
regulated leaves, 90
sick time, 89
time off, 86, 90
unpaid leave, 86
unpaid time off, 54, 88
LPR. *See* Lawful Permanent Resident

M
Making the Offer, 103
background check, 103
reference check, 103
Mayo Clinic, 23

Mentorship, 27
Minimum Wage, 144

N
National Labor Relations Act, 155
NLRA. *See* National Labor Relations Act
Non-Salaried Compensation, 81.
See also salaried compensation

O
Occupational Safety and Health Act of
1970, 154
Occupational Safety and Health Administration, 154
Office of Personnel Management, 60
Onboarding, 95, 103
benefits of well-organized program,
105
five questions from new employee,
104
initial, 106
orientation, 106
strategies to prevent employee
remorse, 105
OPM. *See* Office of Personnel
Management
Organization Objectives, 163
Organizational Culture, 17
Organizational Culture Improvement,
22
strategic benefits, 18
Organizational Design, 58-59
Organizational Overview, 106
Organizing Principles, 66
Orientation, 106
benefits, 106
employee handbook, 107
functions & standards, 109
introduction to workspace, 108
pay & time management, 109
the first 90 days, 110
OSHA. *See* Occupational Safety and
Health Administration